# SOAP AND WATER & COMMON SENSE

SOAP AND WATER & COMMON SENSE

# soap *and* water

# common sense

## THE DEFINITIVE GUIDE TO VIRUSES, BACTERIA, PARASITES, AND DISEASE

## Dr. BONNIE HENRY

ANANSI

First published in 2009 by House of Anansi Press Inc.
This edition published in Canada in 2020
and the USA in 2020 by House of Anansi Press Inc.
www.houseofanansi.com

House of Anansi Press is committed to protecting our natural environment. This book is made of material from well-managed FSC®-certified forests, recycled materials, and other controlled sources.

24 23 22 21 20     1 2 3 4 5

Library and Archives Canada Cataloguing in Publication

Title: Soap and water & common sense : the definitive guide to viruses, bacteria, parasites, and disease / Dr. Bonnie Henry.
Other titles: Soap and water and common sense
Names: Henry, Bonnie, Dr., author.
Identifiers: Canadiana 20200206885 | ISBN 9781487008673 (softcover)
Subjects: LCSH: Communicable diseases—History. |
LCSH: Communicable diseases—Prevention. |
LCSH: Communicable diseases—Transmission. | LCSH: Hygiene.
Classification: LCC RC113 .H46 2020 | DDC 616.909—dc23

Cover image: Zara Ronchi/Getty Images

 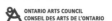

We acknowledge for their financial support of our publishing program the Canada Council for the Arts, the Ontario Arts Council, and the Government of Canada.

Printed and bound in Canada

In memory of Dr. Sheela Basrur,
my mentor, friend, and partner in public health.
You are deeply missed.

And for my mentor Perry Kendall

# CONTENTS

# CONTENTS

# INTRODUCTION TO THE
# NEW EDITION

IN JUNE 2003, at the midpoint of the SARS epidemic, I visited my sister, Dr. Bonnie Henry, on the eleventh floor of the public-health building in downtown Toronto, Canada, where she was leading the city's operational response under the direction of the extraordinary, empathetic, and impressive Dr. Sheela Basrur. Almost two decades later, I can still see in my mind's eye one particular scene: my sister leading me through a warren of cubicles and offices into a hushed, windowless boardroom, where we paused for a few minutes while she consulted urgently with colleagues. Left on my own for a moment, my eyes were drawn to the far wall, which featured a whiteboard bristling from end to end with Post-it Notes of various colours, connected by thin unbroken lines of black ink. As I stared at this strangely beautiful abstraction, its meaning slowly came into focus: this was the track of the awful disease itself, and these colours were the stages of its relentless progress within the web of people it had infected.

Today, in mid-March 2020, I sit in the sun (spring still proceeds; the cherry trees still blossom) at my sister's kitchen table in British Columbia, Canada, in the messy middle of a far more extensive worldwide pandemic whose full shape and range and effect we do not yet know — although we understand more every day and scramble to assimilate and disseminate life-saving scraps of knowledge before the unyielding calculus of the disease engulfs us. The memory of the rainbow of notes on that whiteboard haunts me, with its eerie combination of the abstract, precise, and mathematical with the fragile and personal. It occurs to me that we all exist, right now, somewhere as-yet undiscovered on that whiteboard — in the space between those poles of the coolly abstract and the shockingly personal. And we are dependent upon the few who can effectively articulate and traverse that space for us, with us, and hopefully one small step ahead of us.

Now, ten years after the publication of the first edition of *Soap and Water & Common Sense*, Dr. Bonnie Henry has emerged as one of the most influential, calm, and compassionate voices tracing the precipitous, dizzying curve of the COVID-19 pandemic in (at the time of this writing) almost-daily press conferences. I stole a few minutes from her nearly impossible schedule to ask her two questions for this updated edition of the book.

LYNN HENRY: Bonnie, in my lifetime and yours we have lived through AIDS, SARS, Ebola, and H1N1, to name but a few infectious diseases that have affected large populations. Yet today we seem to be dealing with something that has no precedent in living memory, at least where pandemics are concerned. Do you think the COVID-19 pandemic is different and, if so, why and how?

DR. BONNIE HENRY: Well, as you know, I have been studying the transmission of disease nationally and internationally for decades. I've sat on many, many public-health committees in Canada and worldwide and attended countless conferences and gatherings. I've participated in studying the modelling of infectious disease and in drafting numerous responses and plans for outbreaks. But I will be completely honest: I just never, ever, ever thought I would have to do what I am doing right now [declaring a state of emergency to deal with the COVID-19 pandemic in my home province of British Columbia].

Why is this different? Is it really different? Well, yes and no. COVID-19 is not dissimilar to AIDS and Ebola in terms of the fear it generates, although I would suggest that the sense of fear for one's personal physical health around both of those diseases was perhaps greater — especially among those who contracted either of them, and in their early stages. AIDS was, for a time, equivalent to a death sentence. And of course, that fact generated other terrible and destructive fears beyond the physical. The same was, and is, true in a somewhat different fashion with Ebola. But the difference between those two diseases and COVID-19 has to do with the means of transmission: this new coronavirus spreads through droplets in the air, which makes it a far greater unknown and instills in us a sense that we have no individual control over whether or not we come in contact with it. We cannot see its pathway with the naked eye, and the behavioural controls we can exercise involve not just us, but our entire communities (as we are seeing in the lockdowns of countries at this moment and the practice of so-called social distancing). To know that we can get sick simply by the basic, necessary act of breathing itself — something that is true with COVID-19 but not with AIDS and Ebola — means that of course we are fearful.

When we look at SARS and influenza, we see that in one way COVID-19 is not so different. Those diseases, too, can spread through droplets in the air. But COVID-19 has that perfect storm of qualities: it is far more infectious than SARS, and it is more lethal than influenza. Add to this the fact that we have never before been more physically connected than we are now, with far greater global community interaction, and we arrive at the very moment we are living through.

LYNN HENRY: It has been ten years since the original publication of *Soap and Water & Common Sense*. We know that there have been advances in certain diseases since 2009, so of course some of the information has changed a bit, and that there have been setbacks in some areas and with some diseases, too — an alarming rise in TB in some places, for example. But is there anything you would change or add to the basic advice and public health tenets you cover in this book? I ask this being mindful especially of our current moment, when people worldwide are isolating to try to "flatten the curve" of the new pandemic.

DR. BONNIE HENRY: Perhaps it seems a little odd to say, but William Osler's words from more than a century ago remain true and are, if anything, more relevant than ever: "Soap and water and common sense are the best disinfectants." I would perhaps expand or amend the basic rules just a little, to say:

- Clean your hands (whether with soap and water, or with alcohol-based hand rubs).

- Cover your mouth when you cough (preferably not with your hand; use your elbow or a tissue instead).

- Avoid touching your face, especially your mouth, nose, and eyes.

- Stay at home and away from others when you are sick.

- And during this time of community disease transmission, rigorously practice social distancing (staying at least two metres away from other people).

I would also add one further life-enhancing daily practice, something that we can all do, and that will undoubtedly save us in troubling times: let us all show kindness and awareness and compassion.

— Lynn Henry and Dr. Bonnie Henry, March 2020

"...what we learn in times of pestilence: that there
are more things to admire in men than to despise."
— Albert Camus, *The Plague*


"If you can't explain it simply,
you don't understand it well enough."
—Albert Einstein

# MICROBES INC.

MICROBES INC.

# ONE

## GOOD BUGS,
## BAD BUGS

THE DOCTOR QUICKLY scanned the chart as she opened the door to the examining room. It was a busy day, and the patient had been squeezed into her schedule. The new mom with the crying infant on her lap looked harried and tired. The baby had developed a fever overnight, was clearly irritable, and looked unwell. His mother had tried some medication to relieve the fever but was certain the child had developed another ear infection and needed antibiotics. Feeling the pressure of the crowded waiting room and knowing she was already at least a half-hour behind schedule, the doctor hesitated. Her instincts told her the baby had probably caught a virus and the symptoms would resolve on their own in a day or two. But the child's mother was insistent; she couldn't take another sleepless night of worry.

This dilemma is faced every day by doctors around the world. With our overburdened health-care systems, taking the time to reassure patients and explain why antibiotics won't work is difficult for many health professionals to do. It is far easier and takes less precious time to succumb to the demand for antibiotics. These powerful medications have been available for only a few decades, and they have earned their reputation as "miracle drugs" by saving people from infections that used to kill. But the fact that they are effective only against bacteria — not viruses — has been lost in the excitement. We now know that the overuse and misuse of these miracle drugs are having long-term effects on our precious medical defences and are putting our health at risk. If only people knew the difference.

❀

EVERY DAY, THE media inundate us with medical stories covering everything from miracle drugs to superbugs. In addition, we are bombarded with aggressive advertising campaigns from drug companies that tout medications promising to cure whatever ails us. It's nearly impossible to separate fact from fiction. Understanding how we get sick and what causes those nasty infections can help.

This book will navigate you through the complex world of bugs — those that cause illness and also those that play a role in keeping us healthy. We will cover the myths and misconceptions your doctor doesn't always have time to explain, and we will explore why the fundamental differences between viruses, bacteria, fungi, and parasites are important to our health. We will demystify the complex world of drugs, and we will look at the fascinating history of vaccines, antibiotics, and other measures that have been developed to protect us from some of the worst culprits in the ever-changing microbe world. We will explore the world of superbugs, and show how our actions can contribute to making these bugs so much more dangerous. We will lay naked the bug and expose its inner workings, and we will look at the three simple rules that can help us stay healthy: clean your hands, cover your mouth when you cough, and stay at home when you have a fever. Dr. William Osler's words ring as true today as they did more than a hundred years ago: "Soap and water and common sense are the best disinfectants."

## MICROBES INCORPORATED

Thousands of people get sick from diseases caused by micro-organisms that we inadvertently pick up from contaminated surfaces, ingest in our food, or inhale from the air. Countless hours of misery are caused by bugs called viruses, bacteria, fungi, and parasites — yet much of this suffering is preventable.

Welcome to the awe-inspiring world of Microbes Inc., a global corporation that has dominated our planet for three billion years. As in any global conglomerate, there are several divisions in the world of bugs, or microbes, and while they can all cause illness, some can be beneficial too. Let's take a tour through the halls of Microbes Inc. and explore the different divisions.

### Viruses

The first group of bugs is the smallest and often the most lethal: the viruses. Viruses are small packets of genetic material that have evolved over billions of years to infect humans, animals, and even plants; no living organism can escape from the destructive touch of viruses. Viruses need to use another organism's cells in order to replicate and survive. They reproduce by inserting themselves into the cells of the body, where they hijack the programming mechanism that the cells use to replicate, making thousands and thousands of copies of themselves instead. The replicated viruses then burst out into the bloodstream, killing the initial infected cell and sending the legions of copies to find and infect more cells.

Viruses can cause illness by destroying human cells in a matter of hours or days, and they have been the cause of some of the most frightening and deadly diseases we know. And because viruses are made up of such small pieces of genetic material, they can change or mutate rapidly and have perfected this skill to evade our best efforts at containing them.

Human genetic material, or genes, consists of two strands of deoxyribonucleic acid, or DNA: the fascinating double helix that was first discovered by Nobel Prize–winning scientists James Watson and Francis Crick. This discovery revolutionized our understanding of how human genes replicate and how they determine everything from our hair and eye colour to whether we will develop diseases like cancer or Parkinson's. DNA is formed when two strands of ribonucleic acid (RNA) match in very specific ways. Each strand of RNA is composed of basic building blocks called bases, which are strung together in very specific patterns. There are four types of bases: adenine (A), cytosine (C), guanine (G), and thymine (T). Pairs of bases form a pattern that determines how the gene will be expressed in the person. So whether you will have blue eyes or brown eyes depends on how the RNA strands match up. If just one base is out of place or replaced, it can lead to very different outcomes.

It turns out that bugs have the same type of genetic material as humans, with the exception of a whole family of viruses, the RNA viruses, which have only a single strand of genetic material, or RNA. So while humans and DNA viruses have a double-checking mechanism for every time they replicate, the RNA viruses lack this biological trait. This means that the RNA viruses can reproduce much more quickly and are much more likely to introduce coding errors (like a base out of place) while they are replicating. We call this phenomenon "mutation."

Some mutations can affect the virus's ability to infect cells. These viruses die out quickly because they can no longer replicate their genetic material. But every now and then a mutation will come along that allows the virus to increase its rate of infection of new cells or hosts or to work around any defences we have developed (such as vaccines or antibodies). These mutations can open up whole new worlds to the virus's destructive power.

About five thousand viruses are known and have been characterized, but there are probably a hundred times more that we have not yet encountered. Let's look at a few viruses that have caused some of the most frightening illnesses known to humankind.

*Smallpox*
Throughout history the diseases caused by viruses have disrupted nations and destroyed everything from livestock to food supplies to entire communities. In the world of Microbes Inc. the senior VP of the virus department would have to be smallpox. Until the disease was eradicated in 1979, smallpox caused untold suffering for at least a thousand years in communities around the world. The smallpox virus invaded the cells of the skin, causing large, painful blisters that burst open, spewing highly contagious fluids and leaving the sufferer

scarred for life. Tombs of ancient Egyptian kings are engraved with images of people marked by smallpox scars. The disease is also known to have decimated Native populations across North America. One of our greatest medical achievements has been the removal of this scourge from the planet.

## SARS

The 2003 SARS (severe acute respiratory syndrome) outbreak is a perfect example of the havoc a virus can wreak around the globe. This ambitious upstart probably emerged from the untimely mixing of two or more rather tame viruses in wild animals, leading to mutations that enabled the new virus to infect humans. Scientists worldwide scrambled to track the origins of this deadly new bug, which spread suddenly and rapidly between people, causing severe influenza-like symptoms that could quickly lead to death. The bug was first detected in southern Guangdong Province in China in November 2002. But because the Chinese government for several months denied any outbreak of disease, this new and dangerous bug was given a timely head start. It managed to reach Hong Kong in February 2003, hitchhiking in the lungs of a doctor from Guangzhou, the province's capital, and within days had started its destructive journey to countries around the world. Over the next six months SARS spread from Hong Kong to Singapore to Vietnam to Taiwan to Beijing and Toronto.

This fascinating journey was carefully pieced together by epidemiologists, the microbe hunters of the medical world, who determined that the origin of the virus was in the "wet markets" of Guangdong Province. There a harmless coronavirus that caused mild sickness in some animals, but not humans, somehow managed to acquire a new piece of genetic material that allowed it to greatly expand its infecting universe. Testing of animals in the area where the SARS virus first emerged indicates that the bug probably got its start in wild civet cats that were raised in cages in the local wet markets and later served at restaurants. From the markets of Guangzhou the virus spread to Hong Kong, and with the help of travellers it continued to spread to cities around the world. The SARS story is truly a reflection of our modern mobile society.

## Ebola

Ebola, another relatively new hire at Microbes Inc., is a virus that invades the blood, organs, and even layers of the skin, causing its victim to bleed everywhere, from the lining of their eyes to their intestines. The virus was named after the Ebola River in Zaire (now Democratic Republic of the Congo), where it first drew international attention in 1976 for decimating the village of Yambuku, affecting four hundred villagers and Belgian missionaries.

The Ebola virus was still very much an enigma in 1995, when another massive outbreak invaded Kikwit, Zaire. The people of Zaire had withstood decades of corruption and greed under the ruthless dictatorship of Mobutu Sese Seko, who had exploited the nation's vast mineral wealth and left the country with severe food shortages, a complete lack of infrastructure, a health system in tatters, and the highest child mortality rates in the world. In this tragic setting where people were used to seeing the young die of disease, starvation, or military assault, the gruesome nature of Ebola left even those who had seen so much suffering in despair.

Ebola is a virus that preys on acts of compassion, infecting those who nurse the sick or care for the bodies of the dead. The bug spread easily between patients and the few health-care workers in the rudimentary hospital, where basic infection-control measures such as handwashing were not in effect. The Kikwit outbreak was contained through the heroic efforts of the international medical community, particularly experts from the World Health Organization (WHO) and Médicins Sans Frontières, who worked with the traumatized local community. But it was not gone for long.

Despite intensive efforts to understand the workings of this devastating disease, the world was still unprepared when the next major outbreak hit the town of Gulu, Uganda, in 1999–2000. We still do not know where the virus lay dormant between these outbreaks, but many scientists suspect that local bats may have played a role. In addition, there is no effective treatment for the disease, although a vaccine is in development, and no effective early warning system to detect the active virus and prevent its spread in high-risk areas. Like many of the top performers of Microbes Inc., Ebola has shown an uncanny ability to find the areas of the world most affected by poverty, war, starvation, and disease and to exploit an already vulnerable population barely clinging to life.

*Influenza*
Influenza, another senior manager at Microbes Inc., is a bug that has been credited as being the number-one killer of human populations. Circling the globe annually, this virus preys on the young and the elderly, leading to thousands of deaths worldwide every year. Because this virus has only one strand of nuclear material (RNA), it can change rapidly and takes on new bits of genetic material as quickly as it can. Every year the influenza virus changes just enough that the human immune system no longer recognizes it, and new immunization must be developed to combat the new form of flu. But the virus can also change in a major way at short

notice, leading to major pandemics, or worldwide outbreaks of disease. In the past century and a half, a major global outbreak of influenza has occurred about every forty years. A pandemic is a disease that circles the world, affecting people in many countries. This is in contrast to an epidemic or an outbreak, which are the terms used for diseases that cause illness in smaller areas. There have been three influenza pandemics in the past century, but the "Spanish flu" of 1918–19 still stands out as the most devastating pandemic in world history.

In the past decade, the emergence in Southeast Asia and China of new variants of "avian" or "bird" influenza viruses has captured the attention of the world medical community. It has even led to the World Health Organization's urgent pleading for countries around the globe to plan for the next influenza pandemic — all this for a virus strain that has proven lethal to chickens but has yet to pass successfully between people. The unfortunate few who have contracted the disease have died at a much higher rate than those infected by the more common influenza strains that we have seen in the past forty years. In addition, the avian flu virus has made victims of the young and robust, those whose immune systems are not usually as vulnerable to infection. It may be only a matter of time before this adaptable bug manages to find a way to transmit efficiently between people through an innocent cough or sneeze and spread around the world.

While the world was watching Southeast Asia and the avian influenza bug, another virus quietly emerged in Mexico City in mid-April 2009. Hospital staff began reporting severe pneumonia in many young people, some of whom were rapidly dying. Samples were sent to the National Microbiology Laboratory in Canada, and within days a new influenza virus had been identified as the cause.

H1N1 influenza A virus had emerged again, but this time the bug had acquired new pieces of genetic material from swine in Europe and North America and mixed them with some human flu genes. By the time the bug was recognized, this virus had already adapted to the human system and was passing easily between people through coughing and sneezing. Within a week, hundreds of people in the United States and Canada and throughout Mexico had contracted this new form of influenza, and sporadic cases were showing up in Europe and South America. The WHO raised its pandemic alert level from three to five, the second-highest ranking on the scale used to indicate how close we are to a full-blown global pandemic. Outside of Mexico the cases seemed to be mild, more in keeping with seasonal influenza, but countries around the world stepped up their monitoring systems and continue to watch this bug closely. If we have learned one thing about the influenza virus, it is just how unpredictable this bug can be.*

### HIV

Another relative newcomer to Microbes Inc. that has had a spectacular long-term impact on the world's health is the human immunodeficiency virus or HIV. This RNA virus likely emerged in Africa sometime in the early 1980s, though scientists have since discovered the virus in human blood samples dating from at least three decades earlier.

HIV invades the cells of the human immune system, where it hides out patiently, sometimes for many years, before becoming active. The virus then attacks the cells in the human body that defend against infections, leaving the patient vulnerable to severe illnesses that those with healthy immune systems are able to fight off. AIDS, or acquired

---

* This section was written in the early stages of the 2009 influenza pandemic and reflects what was known at the time.

immune deficiency syndrome, is the medical term used to describe the stage of illness when HIV has compromised the immune system and these infections start to take hold. AIDS-defining illnesses include severe progressive tuberculosis, *Pneumocystis carinii* pneumonia, candida, cytomegalovirus infection, and a rare form of cancer called Kaposi's sarcoma. It can take many years before HIV leads to AIDS, because of the discovery of medications that suppress the virus. But there is still no cure for HIV, and once AIDS manifests its effects on the body, it will lead to certain death.

While HIV has undoubtedly devastated many families and communities, it has also been a major force in bringing together governments and health organizations to re-evaluate infection prevention and control measures. The disease has also spawned a whole specialization in medicine that deals only with the complexities of the virus. Beyond the medical system, HIV/AIDS has affected the economy, demographics, and social structure of families, communities, and entire countries, particularly in Africa, which has been disproportionately affected by this malignant bug.

❊

THESE ARE JUST a few of the many bugs that make up the Virus Division of Microbes Inc. Many more viruses will appear in the following chapters, but for now let's take the stairs to the next floor and have a look at a group of bugs that is not all bad. In fact, we probably couldn't live without them.

## Bacteria

The next floor up in the headquarters of Microbes Inc. contains the bugs in the Bacteria Division. Whereas viruses are made up of small packets of genetic material, bacteria are single-celled organisms shaped like rods, spheres, and spirals that have the capacity to reproduce indefinitely and independently, provided they have sufficient nutrients and a suitable environment — such as the human body. Some even have the capacity to change into a spore- or seed-like form, building a protective wall that is highly resistant to destruction. These bacterial spores, which are produced by bugs such as anthrax and *Clostridium*, can survive for decades in even the harshest environments. When conditions improve, they re-emerge, becoming active and causing disease. A classic example is the large outbreak of anthrax in cattle in Saskatchewan, Canada, in 2006, after record rainfall and flooding provided an ideal environment for the spores to emerge. Anthrax hadn't caused disease in that part of the Prairies for close to fifty years, but the spores had waited patiently in the soil until the conditions were just right. The bacteria then spread to the vulnerable cattle, crippling the Saskatchewan beef industry.

Bacteria, like humans, have DNA. Unlike viruses, bacteria are not dependent on the genetic apparatus of other cells to reproduce, and they can acquire new DNA in several ways. The first and most common way bacteria exchange bits of DNA is through merging, or microbe sex. Bacteria can reproduce at an astounding rate, producing millions of generations in a matter of hours (compare this to the human reproduction process, which takes somewhere around fifteen years to produce a generation). In addition, the new bacteria may pick up a piece of DNA that allow them to resist antibiotics, so the bug can live longer (survival of the fittest, at a micro level) and in many cases become stronger.

Bacteria can also acquire new DNA by swallowing up or ingesting bits of genetic material from the DNA of dead bacteria in their environment. This form of reproduction is completely foreign to humans, or any other multicellular organism, and gives the bacteria an incredible survival advantage. This ability to ingest the DNA of dead bacteria explains why a patient unfortunate enough to be infected with two bacteria at the same time can suddenly develop resistance to antibiotics.

The third way bacteria acquire new genetic matter hints at the complex interactions between the divisions at Microbes Inc. Viruses have the ability to infect bacteria by inserting a little piece of their own genetic material into the bacterial DNA. This process can lead to the evolution of the infected bacteria. But the virus can also take a chunk of the bacterium's DNA when it leaves the cell and transpose this genetic material to other bacteria, spreading the word, as it were, even farther.

In terms of sheer numbers, bacteria are the most successful organisms on the planet, and they have adapted to live in every environment imaginable. These bugs can live and thrive in everything from pools of sulphur to completely oxygen-free air to the boiling water of deep-sea volcanoes and everything in between. Bacteria are also one of our biggest natural energy sources, since they can process just about every type of substance in existence. Some species have even developed the ability to feed on and thereby break down plastics.

Bacteria are a natural part of the human condition: we live in a soup of bacteria both in and on our bodies and in our environment. Some estimates suggest that we have more than 100,000 individual bacteria per square centimetre on our skin! But unlike viruses, not all bacteria are bad bugs. We depend on bacteria for many things, from helping us digest milk to the production of yogurt, cheese, and other foods like fermented cabbage (sauerkraut and kimchee) and soy sauce. In addition, these "good bugs"—our "normal flora," as we affectionately call these bacteria in the medical world—help us to achieve a balance within our human systems, and they are tolerated by our immune systems without making us sick.

"Bad bugs," or infectious bacteria, on the other hand, replicate beyond the well-being of their host, causing illness and sometimes death. This can happen for a variety of reasons; for example, the bacteria on our skin may pick up a piece of DNA that allows them to resist antibiotics. This often happens in a hospital setting, where a patient who has been on antibiotics for a long time can pass on to other people a bacterial strain that has evolved to resist those medications. The antibiotic-resistant bacteria can be passed along by the contaminated hands of health-care workers or from innocently touching a washroom door in a hospital room shared by four patients. Either way, these new antibiotic-resistant bacteria have developed an evolutionary advantage, defying our usual antibiotic treatment and making the infection much more difficult to deal with. This process has led to the development of the so-called superbug, which we will review in the next chapter. For now, let's look more closely at some of the main bacterial players, particularly those that can cause illness and disease.

### Staphylococcus and Streptococcus

Many of the offices in the Bacteria Division are occupied by *Staphylococcus* and *Streptococcus*. Strains of these two long-time leaders have made their homes on human skin and in our mouths and throats. Our skin acts as a waterproof barrier that protects us from getting infections. Having these normal bacteria on the skin's surface helps our bodies function and maintain a fine balance.

When the skin is broken, our immune system is tested, and that is when our normal flora can cause problems. Most commonly these take the form of skin infections, or cellulitis, and small pustules or abscesses. If our immune system is run down, say after receiving chemotherapy treatment for cancer or recovering from a bad viral infection, both *Staphylococcus* and *Streptococcus* can cause more severe, even deadly infections such as pneumonia (infection of the lungs) or sepsis (infection of the blood, or "blood poisoning").

*Tuberculosis*
*Mycobacterium tuberculosis*, or TB, is the senior VP of the Bacteria Division, having spent centuries infecting and killing people all over the world and from all walks of life. The disease has gone by many names over the centuries, including the White Death and consumption. From kings and queens to writers and painters, TB has led to the premature death of some of our most famous citizens.

This bacterium most often invades the lungs but can affect every part of the body from the bones to the lymph nodes to the brain. It can also remain dormant in the body for years before becoming active and unleashing its destructive force. The classic symptoms caused by this bug are blood-tinged cough from infection in the lungs, weight loss, and fatigue. In months, sometimes years, people are "consumed" by the bug until they no longer have the strength to breathe.

TB was temporarily thwarted in much of the Western world by improved sanitation and general nutrition, plus the development of antibiotics in the 1950s. But the bacterium has made a dramatic resurgence, and new strains of the disease have proven resistant to treatment. Couple this terrible bug with HIV, and even more severe illness develops more rapidly in the human host. This deadly duo is decimating families and destroying the way of life of entire communities and even countries. The effects of TB and HIV are particularly devastating in sub-Saharan Africa, where tuberculosis is the number-one cause of death by infectious disease and access to treatment may be several days' walk away or, in many places, non-existent.

## Cholera

Another ancient disease that has made a comeback in recent decades is the scourge of cholera. Cholera is caused by a bacterium called *Vibrio cholerae*, which kills by essentially draining the body of water. The bug attaches to the lining of the intestines and hijacks the cells that regulate the amount of water we absorb and the amount we excrete as waste in the stool. When things are working well, we take in more water than we pass out. Water is essential for just about all our body functions and is the main component of most of our cells from blood to skin. Cholera bugs press the "excrete" button in every intestinal cell, stopping any absorption and causing a loss of 25 percent of body weight in mere hours. Death comes in as little as twenty-four hours unless the fluid is replaced rapidly and in large volumes.

Cholera is passed between people by what we call the "fecal-oral" route. The bug is most often transmitted from water or food contaminated with human excrement. Once in a new host, the bacterium settles in the intestines and rapidly reproduces until the body gives out. In some cases the immune system is able to rescue the patient from this terminal fate. The natural evolutionary pattern of all bugs is to weaken a person for long enough that the bug can reproduce and pass its legacy generation on to another host. It is in this way that the species survives.

Cholera outbreaks were documented in Sanskrit writings as far back as 500 B.C. For centuries the disease was confined largely to India and the Asian subcontinent, but by the mid 1800s cholera had found its nirvana in the densely populated cities of Europe and the United Kingdom, where the chances of finding a new host to infect were suddenly increased exponentially. Whether it was because of extreme overcrowding or inadequate — in some cases truly primitive — sewer systems that connected with drinking-water supplies, cholera no longer had to wait for victims; they were there for the taking. The bacteria could also make people deathly ill in a matter of hours because it was assured that the bug's progeny would inevitably find a new host to infect. Once improved sanitation and safe drinking-water systems were introduced into the city's infrastructure, cholera outbreaks became rare again, except in its ancient homes on the Asian subcontinent.

But the story doesn't end there. Ever seeking new ways to secure its survival, the cholera bug bided its time, causing small outbreaks in communities in India and Bangladesh while continually evolving to adapt to new conditions. Then when global travel and trade increased in the 1980s and 1990s, the bacterium found a chance to strike again. Hitchhiking in the bowels of ocean-going ships that carried goods from India to South America, cholera found a new home in Peru in 1991 when the vessels pumped their ballast into the harbour.

South America hadn't seen cholera for more than a hundred years (the last outbreak was in 1895) when this new strain, called El Tor, arrived on its shores. Through lack of hygiene the disease spread from street vendors selling contaminated seafood and beverages with contaminated ice. From Peru this new strain of cholera spread rapidly to Brazil, El Salvador, Nicaragua, Honduras, Guatemala, Mexico, Bolivia, Ecuador, and Colombia, leaving more than one million people sick and over ten thousand deaths in its wake in just five years. The economic loss to Peru alone cost the country US$495 billion.

The world of Microbes Inc. thus taught us another lesson: never be complacent. Complacency can be costly, and deadly.

## Fungi: Moulds and Yeasts

The third major division of Microbes Inc. is a mixed group of single- and multi-celled bugs called fungi. The members of this division are varied and their effects on humans, animals, and plants are equally as different, though for the most part less severe than those of their bacteria and virus colleagues. In many ways they are the workhorses of Microbes Inc., adding all sorts of good things to the world and now and then causing some havoc. The most important types of fungi that can affect our health are the single-celled yeasts and the multi-celled moulds.

Moulds and yeasts have strong protective cell walls made of a protein substance called chitin, which allows these bugs to survive in some very unusual environments. More independent than their bacteria and virus co-workers, moulds and yeasts reproduce on their own, sometimes forming long filaments, or hyphae (think of an old piece of bread with furry green mould). Fungi have more complex DNA than viruses or bacteria and can grow to be quite large, large enough to be seen by the human eye. Mushrooms and truffles are examples of fungi that most of us are familiar with. They are by far the largest members of this group of more than 1.5 million species.

Fungi, especially moulds and yeasts, play many roles in our world, from decomposing organic matter (along with bacteria) to causing fermentation to providing valuable sources of medications. They can also produce toxins that are particularly lethal to humans. One potent toxin, called aflatoxin, is produced by a fungus that affects peanuts; even a minute amount of this substance can be lethal if ingested. Yet it is difficult to imagine our world without these bugs. Yeast is essential to the production of wine and beer and for baking bread, while a mould called *Aspergillus* yields tempeh and soy sauce. Another produces the "blue" in cheeses such as Stilton and Roquefort. In addition, these good bugs are the source of a number of bacteria-killing agents called antibiotics; from them we have developed drugs such as the penicillins and cephalosporins. Most human illnesses caused by fungi (mostly yeasts or moulds) tend to be relatively mild — conditions such as ringworm, skin infections, and athlete's foot — but some have more serious results and can even be deadly.

*Cryptococcus Mystery*
*Cryptococcus gattii* is a modern example of how lethal a fungus can be. This rare yeast lives in soil and the bark of certain trees, mostly eucalyptus, and has been present in areas of Africa, Australia, and southern California for decades. In 1999 it managed to get a toehold in the rainforests of central Vancouver Island in British Columbia, Canada, an area of the

world where it had never been seen before. The bug may have been introduced to the region in ballast dumped by ships from Asia; we may never really know. Once on land, this fungus found a suitable home in local trees. Whether because of global warming or just plain luck, the bug was able to thrive and spread explosively over the next eight years, leading to infections in people who inhaled the yeast cells or spores. By 2007 *Cryptococcus gattii* had caused more than 216 people to fall ill with pneumonia, weight loss, night sweats, and fevers, and was responsible for at least eight deaths. Like many members of Microbes Inc., the bug preys on people with weakened immune systems. So while several thousand people may have been exposed to the fungus, only a relative few fell severely ill. This nasty bug is treatable with a potent antifungal medicine, but it took some time before public health disease trackers were able to identify the yeast and educate doctors, who were assessing patients with lung infections. For some it was too late.

*The Great Potato Famine*
Perhaps the most well-known fungus in history is a bug that doesn't make humans ill but in some ways changed the face of the world. This fungus goes by the grand Latin name *Phytophthora infestans* but is known the world over as potato blight. This bug was the cause of the great Irish potato famine from 1845 to 1849. The fungus was known in its time as potato cholera for the terrible smell it caused in the rotting spuds. The effects of this bug led to the death of 1.5 million people over five years and the exodus of millions of Irish peasants to the shores of North America.

The Irish potato blight is a cautionary tale that we need to heed even today. In 1533 potatoes were imported to Spain from Peru, and the crop had spread to the rest of Europe by early 1600. The original Andean species were hardy tubers that resisted pests such as potato blight. Over time its genetic diversity, which protected the plant in the wild, was bred out of the potato to offer consumers a more pleasing, uniform product. Unfortunately the potato was then no longer able to defend itself against disease.

When potato blight spread to Ireland in 1845, it found fields and fields of susceptible hosts ripe for attack. The population was dependent upon the plant for their diet, and potato cholera led to the starvation of millions of people. This same issue of overbreeding has also resulted in ruined banana crops in Ecuador and widespread disease in vineyards in France. While a single uniform plant product may be beneficial to markets and trade, it creates a weakened species susceptible to the destructive forces of many bad bugs and can have a far-reaching effect on the health of our societies.

## Parasites

Members of the final division of Microbes Inc. are the largest in size but have roles as diverse as many of their colleagues. Parasites are bugs that derive nourishment and protection from other living organisms, known as hosts. Many of them find the human body to be the perfect host for some or all of their life cycle. They range in size from microscopic single-cell bugs that are ten times larger than bacteria to multicellular creatures that can be seen with the naked eye. Tapeworms are a good example of larger parasites; some can even grow to be six metres long.

Parasites can be transmitted from animals to humans, from humans to humans, and even from humans to animals.

These bugs live and reproduce in the tissue and organs of infected hosts and are often excreted as hardy spores or eggs in the feces. They are known to be the cause of food- and water-borne illness around the world, and some of the smaller and more devastating members use vectors such as mosquitoes to find their next victim.

About 70 percent of parasites are one-celled bugs. *Giardia* is a common parasite that lives in rivers and streams and forms a hardy cyst that can easily survive the body's digestive juices. When ingested, the bug infects the intestines, causing nasty stomach cramps and diarrhea. Another one-celled parasite is *Toxoplasma gondii*, a unique bug that carries out its reproductive cycle in members of the cat family. In its infective phase the bug forms a strong cyst called an oocyst, which is shed into the environment in cat feces. In its quest to find a new cat to invade, it can sometimes be ingested by humans. While toxoplasmosis rarely makes cats ill, the parasite can cause fevers, swollen lymph nodes, and muscle aches in humans, and those with weakened immune systems can experience permanent eye and brain damage.

The other 30 percent of workers in the Parasite Division are large multicellular bugs we can see with the naked eye. They include roundworms, pinworms, hookworms, tapeworms, and flukes. The preferred hosts for most of these bugs are the animals we rely on for food. They are especially adept at spreading between domesticated cattle and swine that are bred in large, crowded farms. While improved animal husbandry practices in much of the Western world have limited the range of these bugs, their influence is still great in many countries and has had an impact on everything from our food sources to religious practices.

*Malaria*

The most famous member of the Parasite Division is the one-celled bug called *Plasmodium*, which causes the deadly disease malaria. This remarkable bug has survived for centuries, adapting to just about every place on earth and resisting attempts to contain the disease. Malaria is one of the most influential diseases in human history, and while its impact is no longer felt in much of northern Europe and North America it is still prevalent in Southeast Asia and is responsible for killing as many as a million children a year in Africa.

The history of malaria is the history of man's interface with nature. When humans began farming some six thousand years ago, contact was made with insect species that were previously isolated in the forests. One of the key new contacts was mosquitoes. There are several thousand species of mosquitoes, and about 10 percent transmit diseases to humans. Mosquitoes are amazingly opportunistic, and several species have adapted to survive in specific temperatures, altitudes, and breeding conditions. Some have even adapted to become fully urbanized city dwellers and are able to exist only in the man-made world.

Initially malaria was caused by *Plasmodium ovale*, a species of the bug that produced relatively mild disease in humans. But as we moved farther into mosquito habitat, more virulent strains of the disease emerged. Today the most serious and often deadly infections are caused by *Plasmodium falciparum*, a bug that is now responsible for 95 percent of deaths caused by malaria. This parasite has had such a devastating effect on populations in Africa that people in the area have developed a genetic adaptation called sickle-cell trait, which protects them against the disease. Yet despite our best defences, this pesky parasite continues to have a devastating impact on communities around the world.

| DIVISION | SIZE/CHARACTER | PICTURE |
|---|---|---|
| *Viruses* | 100 nanometres (100 billionth of an inch) Uses other organism's cells to reproduce | |
| *Bacteria* | 10 times larger than viruses (at least 1 micron or 4 millionths of an inch) Single-celled microbes that reproduce independently | o |
| *Single-celled parasites, yeast, and fungi* | 10 times larger than bacteria or 0.01 mm Have hard cell walls or form cysts to survive | O |
| *Multicellular parasites* | Can be seen with the naked eye Can be up to 6 m (20 ft) long | ∽ |

HOW DO WE GET SICK?

Microbes have designed many evolutionary strategies to spread to new hosts. They can be inhaled into our lungs, ingested in food and water, exchanged through infected body fluids or absorbed through our skin by direct contact or touch, and finally they can spread through insect and animal bites. It is this innate will to survive that has allowed them to maintain their reign as the dominant species on the planet.

A common way for bugs to spread between humans is through the air. These particular bugs infect a host's respiratory system, forcing the person to cough or sneeze, thus dispelling a moist cloud of microbe mist into the environment that others can easily, and unknowingly, breathe in. These stealthy bugs cause some of the world's most deadly diseases and are the reason why covering your mouth when you cough or sneeze is essential to sparing others from infectious disease.

Other bugs pass through the fecal-oral route, when a host unknowingly ingests the microbes that live in human waste. These microbes spread into the environment by causing diarrhea. Millions of bugs hide out in an infected person's loose, watery stool, and then contaminate food or water that others unknowingly ingest. While this sounds pretty gross, we have to remember that most bugs are microscopic in size; millions and millions of infectious bugs can be living in what appears to be a perfectly clear glass of water. If sanitary conditions are poor or if people do not adequately wash their hands after using the toilet, these bugs can remain active, sometimes for hours, on our hands. And if an infected person handles food for others to consume, the cycle starts again in a new digestive system. This is one of the many reasons why washing your hands or using an alcohol-based hand rub is critical to maintaining good health and stopping the spread of disease.

But disease can also be transmitted through other means such as direct contact or touch. Skin-to-skin contact can spread illness when, for example, an infected pustule on one person touches a small tear in another person's skin. Sexual contact is another common way to transmit disease through direct touch. We can also pass diseases through blood, as we saw so tragically in the 1990s when patients around the world contracted HIV through blood transfusions (this was before policies were instituted that required all blood donations to be tested for the virus). In hospitals and other health-care settings, diseases such as hepatitis B and HIV can be passed on from an accidental needle-stick injury. Bugs are also spread between injection drug users who share tainted equipment. Some can even be transmitted through breast milk or other body secretions such as urine, saliva, or even tears.

Finally there is a whole class of diseases that can be passed on to people by what are known as vectors, the term used for insect, tick, and animal bites. The main culprits in this class are mosquitoes, which are responsible for infecting humans with a nasty range of diseases including malaria, yellow fever, and dengue. With increasing global temperatures these vectors have expanded their reach and now make their homes in areas of the world where the species was previously unknown. The virus that causes dengue, for example, is making a huge comeback in parts of the world that had been free of the bug for decades. Another fearsome bug, passed mainly through bats but also through foxes, raccoons, and dogs, is rabies, a disease that is almost always fatal in humans.

The respiratory and fecal-oral routes are the two most common ways for bugs to infect new human hosts. Interestingly, most microbes have adapted to perfect only one method of transmission. For example, if you happen to eat food contaminated with an influenza virus, it is unlikely to make you sick, because influenza doesn't have the ability to survive the acid environment of your stomach. On the other hand, if you somehow inhale *Salmonella*, a common bacteria in food, the bug probably will have no effect on your health because it has not developed the ability to attach to the lining of your nose or lungs.

With so many ways of contracting disease and so many dangerous, adaptable bugs, the path to protecting ourselves has been complex. But there have been some major medical advances in the past two hundred years. We will examine the battle between bugs and humans in the next chapter.

# TWO

# HUMANS VS.
# MICROBES

MICROBES HAVE HAD millions of years to perfect their attacks on the human body, while our abilities to effectively rebuff their assaults are barely two centuries old. Still, the evolution and advances of science and medicine is as fascinating as the history of Microbes Inc. From public health measures such as improved environmental conditions to the development of wonder drugs such as antibiotics and vaccines, we'll look at the many protective measures and disease-fighting weapons that have helped save millions of lives.

### Quarantine and Typhoid Mary

One of the earliest attempts at preventing exposure to disease was through a measure known as quarantine. Quarantine was first used in the fourteenth century to protect cities from the Black Death, or the plague. The plague is caused by the bacterium *Yersinia pestis*, which affects the lungs and the lymph nodes and leads to severe and deadly pneumonia. Between 1348 and 1359 the Black Death wiped out an estimated 30 percent of Europe's population, as well as a significant percentage of those living in Asia. The word "quarantine" originates from the Venetian *quaranti giorni*, meaning "forty days." Documents in the archives of Dubrovnik in Dalmatia, which date back to 1377, describe how, before entering the city, visitors were forced to spend thirty days in a restricted location (originally on a nearby island) to see if symptoms of the plague would develop. Later the isolation period was prolonged to forty days and thus named "quarantine." Since that time quarantine has been used extensively across Europe and in the United Kingdom to protect people from diseases such as cholera and yellow fever, and most famously for smallpox. The measure was used in North America when immigrant ships landed on the shores of Ellis Island off New York, Grosse-Île in Quebec, and Lawlor's Island in Halifax harbour.

The most famous person in history to be quarantined was a woman who came to be known as Typhoid Mary. Mary Mallon was an Irish immigrant who worked as a cook in New York City in the early 1900s. She was also a healthy carrier of *Salmonella typhi*, the bacterium that causes the severe gastro-intestinal disease called typhoid. While she remained well, she passed the infection to forty-seven people through the food she prepared; three of them died from the disease. The New York Department of Health investigated the outbreak and found her to be a carrier of the bacterium, though she vehemently denied spreading the disease to others. She was sent to a quarantine hospital on North Brother Island for three years.

In 1914 Mary was released from the hospital on the condition that she never work as a cook again, but what was a poor immigrant woman to do? In 1915 she took up her old profession under an assumed name at the Sloane Hospital for Women in New York, and caused illness in twenty-five people. One patient died as a result. The New York Department of Health traced the outbreak to Mary and she was sent back to North Brother Island for good. She died there in 1938.

In Canada quarantine was enforced during the last major outbreak of smallpox, in Montreal in 1946. The measure was used again in 1962, when a young boy, the son of missionaries to Brazil, developed smallpox in Toronto. He had picked up the virus in Brazil and became sick en route to Canada. Luckily most of the city had been immunized against smallpox, so only a few, non-immune contacts required quarantine.

### The Sanitation Movement

Quarantine was a draconian measure used around the world for centuries when there was little else in the disease-prevention armamentarium. Thankfully, by the late 1800s, despite continued controversy about how disease was caused, there emerged a strong force of medical administrators who were convinced that sanitation measures could help keep people well. They lobbied the government to invest in the city's infrastructure, to protect the public's health by building sewers that collected and treated waste without connecting to the drinking-water system, and to construct plants that filtered any bugs that did get into the drinking water. They also advocated for garbage pickup and management, rodent control measures, and prohibition of spitting on public streets.

Couple the sanitation movement with the isolation of ill people, quarantine of well carriers, and improved nutrition, and we have come a long way in protecting ourselves against infections that only a century ago spread rapidly and killed millions. These measures have been critical to the general health of our society, and today the medical community sees outbreaks of certain diseases as an indicator of the breakdown of these basic public health systems. Cholera outbreaks in war-ravaged areas such as Zimbabwe, Sudan, and the Democratic Republic of the Congo, as well as in Russia following the collapse of the Soviet Union, exemplify the breakdown of a community's public health infrastructure. The prevention of cholera is a key example of a battle won in the war against Microbes Inc.

*John Snow and the Scourge of Cholera*
In 1847 to 1848, parts of London were decimated by one of the most severe cholera outbreaks the city had ever seen. A British physician named John Snow decided to investigate the illness, and his work would play a defining role in the battle against the scourge of his era.

Dr. Snow looked closely at who was getting sick, where they were getting sick, and when the illness took hold. This approach was novel then, but these three characteristics — person, place, and time — are considered essential tools in disease investigation today. Snow wanted to understand why this terrible disease would obliterate an entire family in one house but leave untouched the neighbours across the street or living directly next door. He searched for common factors that linked both the sick and the well and drew maps of where these people lived.

During the Victorian era there were two competing theories about how disease was transmitted. In one camp were those who thought illness was spread by a combination of spontaneous generation and bad air or "miasma," and in the other were those who thought specific "contagions" (germs) were somehow passed between people. Snow was firmly in the contagion camp, and he figured that this cholera outbreak was his chance to discredit the miasma theory.

While the senior medical officer of London believed that miasmas were responsible for the outbreak, Snow had another theory about how cholera moved through the city. He was certain that the drinking-water supply had something to do with the transmission of the disease. Following the 1847–48 outbreak, he patiently mapped out the drinking-water suppliers in his area of London. He knew that some suppliers brought water in to the local neighbourhood pumps from areas in the middle of the Thames River — the same areas where many of the city's sewer systems emptied. Other suppliers brought water from farther up the Thames, away from the main city area. He was sure that the quality of water had something to do with the spread of this terrible disease.

In 1854 another cholera outbreak erupted in a nearby neighbourhood. Snow used this opportunity to take samples from the three main water pumps that provided drinking water to the community. Drawing on his previous research, he was certain that the pump on Broad Street would produce water that was cloudy and of poor quality because it came from an area of the river he felt sure was contaminated with sewage. When Snow talked with residents in the neighbourhood, he was surprised to find that they all preferred to use the Broad Street pump because the water had a reputation for being less murky and tasting better than the water from the two other pumps in the neighbourhood. His samples bore out the neighbours' claims: the water from the Broad

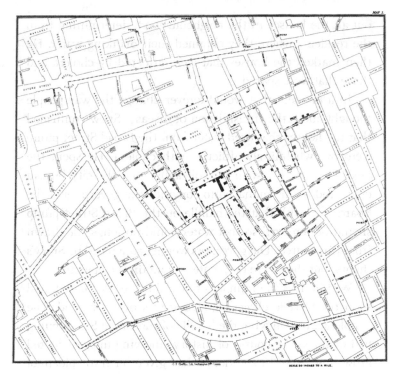

*John Snow's cholera map*

Street pump was much clearer than the water from the other
two pumps.

Snow took the water samples back to his lab to examine
them under his new microscope, a recent invention by
Dutchman Anton van Leeuwenhoek that allowed scientists to
see the tiny bugs in water and other substances. Under the
microscope the water samples told a different story. The water
from the Broad Street pump was literally crawling with microscopic creatures, some of which Snow was sure had something
to do with the spread of cholera. Over the next few days Snow,
assisted by the local clergyman, Henry Whitehead, mapped

out all the houses in the neighbourhood, determining from the residents where they obtained their drinking water. He then marked the houses that were affected by cholera and those that were spared.

In a moment that would forever change the way people thought about the transmission of disease, Snow confirmed that the houses that used water from the Broad Street pump were overwhelmingly afflicted with cholera. He spent the next days arguing with his colleagues and the city bureaucracy and finally managed to convince the governors of the Board of Health that the handle on the Broad Street pump should be removed so that water could no longer be drawn from this source. The governors weren't convinced by Snow's theory, but they were desperate to contain the epidemic.

Within days the number of new illnesses decreased, and soon the terrible cholera epidemic was over for good. The simple act of removing the handle of the Broad Street pump had changed the course of history, allowing unprecedented growth of cities. In addition, it had given birth to epidemiology, a new method of scientific investigation of disease outbreaks that we still use today. Sadly, more than 150 years later cholera is still active in some parts of the world as a result of human conflict and strife, and the enterprising bugs of Microbes Inc. are more than ready to leap into the breach.

### Disease Detectives and World Health

Both quarantine and the sanitation movement soon led to the systematic tracking of contagious disease and the development of public health services around the world. In the late nineteenth century, public health officers adopted a reporting system to monitor diseases, ensure that sanitation systems were working, initiate quarantine if necessary or isolate people who were infectious, and provide vaccination against diseases like smallpox, tuberculosis, or typhoid. But in the beginning public health services were not without controversy.

One of the earliest surveillance systems was developed in New York City in 1897, when the Department of Health made it legally mandatory to document patients who had contracted tuberculosis. Physicians were outraged because the law required them to break the doctor–patient code of confidentiality, which could affect their business and embarrass some prominent members of society. In the end, health officials compromised with the doctors: the names of "dispensary" patients were reported but private patients were not. The Department of Health thought that having at least some information could help to curtail the spread of disease. In reality this meant that the poor were identified but the rich were not, which led to greater stigmatization of the poverty-stricken masses despite the fact that the bug didn't recognize any class distinctions.

Next, legislation was introduced on the surveillance of venereal diseases. The New York City commissioner of health, Dr. Herman Biggs, knew that he was in for an even bigger fight to get doctors onside. He told the Board of Health, "The ten-year-long opposition to the reporting of tuberculosis cases will doubtless appear a mild breeze compared with the stormy protest against the sanitary surveillance of the venereal diseases." It was a fight he eventually won, however, and the first critical step in understanding and controlling disease outbreaks was enacted.

Despite early opposition, surveillance for infectious diseases has become one of the tenets of public health around the world. By 1911, for example, Western Australia had introduced compulsory name-based reporting of all infectious diseases, and in 1915 Sweden made name-based reporting law as well. The Swedish government even went so far as to enact compulsory detention, treatment, and prohibition of marriage for people infected with certain medical conditions such as venereal disease. These measures have been modified over the years and are now less restrictive, but public health authorities must still balance the imposition on an individual's privacy and liberty with protection of our greater society from infectious disease.

As it stands, medical professionals around the world are required by law to report to public health officials the names of patients who have contracted certain diseases. Public health services have also developed the legal and organizational capacity to execute this authority while protecting the confidentiality of the patient. Detecting illness early on can prevent transmission of disease and help contain its spread by measures such as providing medication or vaccine to those already exposed. It also provides valuable information to help epidemiologists monitor trends and detect outbreaks of diseases so measures can be taken to stop them immediately.

## The World Health Organization

The end of the Second World War saw the formation of a global body to monitor diseases. The World Health Organization (WHO) was formed by a resolution of the newly created United Nations on April 7, 1948, which has since become World Health Day. The WHO is governed by the World Health Assembly, which is made up of representatives from countries around the world and sets the direction of the organization. In 1948 the World Health Assembly consisted of fifty-five member countries; today there are 193 members and two associate members.

The WHO provides leadership on matters critical to health by monitoring diseases, assessing trends, and sounding alarms. Initially the organization focused mainly on malaria, tuberculosis, women's and children's health issues (especially immunization), venereal diseases, and environmental sanitation. Many of these issues are as relevant today as they were in 1948. The WHO has led immunization programs in developing countries; alerted the world to outbreaks of Ebola, HIV, and SARS, to name a few; and developed programs regulating food safety and the proper use of medications and vaccines. Much of the critical information we have on infectious disease activity and outbreaks throughout the world, especially in developing countries, comes from the work of epidemiologists and medical disease detectives at the World Health Organization. Epidemiology programs such as the European Centre for Disease Control, the U.S. Centers for Disease Control and Prevention, and many others monitor the health of citizens in their particular jurisdictions and collaborate with the WHO in the fight against Microbes Inc.

The establishment of global public health surveillance and tracking systems and the development of sanitation and safe drinking-water programs remain the underpinning of our work to contain deadly infectious diseases. Added to these infrastructures are measures that help prevent and treat diseases, such as vaccination and medications.

## Vaccination

Following sanitation, hygiene, and the establishment of public health services, the next great discovery in the evolution of disease prevention was vaccination. Vaccination — or as we most commonly refer to it now, immunization — involves priming the immune system with a disease-causing bug by exposing the body to either a killed bug or a piece of the bug's genetic material. The immune system responds by developing antibodies or proteins that remain in the blood. When the body is exposed to the microbe again, the antibodies attack the bug and prevent it from causing illness. This complex process is one of the world's greatest public health achievements and has resulted in protecting societies (particularly children) from some of the most severe and deadly illnesses known to humankind. But the road to effective immunization was long and not without obstacles. It also involved some of the greatest medical and scientific minds in history.

*Edward Jenner and the Milkmaids*
The first major advance in vaccination was the development some two hundred years ago of a vaccine that protected people against the scourge of smallpox. Smallpox claimed hundreds of millions of lives, from Egyptian pharoah Rameses V, who died with telltale scars in 1156 B.C., to a third of the subjects of the Roman Empire during a fifteen-year epidemic around A.D. 165. Millions of Aztec and Inca were devastated by this scourge in the seventeenth century when the disease was introduced into their civilizations by Europeans during the colonization of the Americas. In addition, this bug is infamous for affecting all levels of European society, taking the lives of Queen Mary II of England in 1694, Emperor Joseph I of Austria in 1711, and King Louis XV of France in 1774. In America, President Abraham Lincoln developed smallpox just days after delivering the Gettysburg Address, and George

Washington contracted the disease in 1751 but survived. As well as infecting royalty and political leaders, smallpox ravaged populations worldwide, causing illness, scarring, and death; 10 percent of all fatalities during the eighteenth century were caused by this deadly disease.

Several major smallpox epidemics roared across Europe from the seventeenth to the nineteenth centuries, devastating families and crippling societies. It was in this bleak milieu that an English country doctor first developed the technique we now call vaccination, which has saved millions of lives the world over. Reports as far back as 200 B.C. in ancient China and India document attempts to ward off smallpox by transferring pus or powdered scabs from a mildly infected carrier to a healthy host. But this technique was extremely dangerous and was not widely used during the eighteenth century.

In 1718 Lady Mary Wortley Montagu, wife of the English ambassador to Istanbul and a prolific writer of letters, reported the Turkish practice of "inoculation," in which fluid from a mild case of smallpox was transferred to a healthy host in an attempt to prevent severe disease. Her peers were shocked to learn that she had allowed her infant son to be inoculated, even though it successfully protected him against the disease. She brought knowledge of this practice back to England and the technique spread throughout Europe, mainly among the rich who were able to pay for the procedure. Even the children of the royal family were inoculated, but only after the king first had the procedure tested on six condemned prisoners. The Russian empress Catherine the Great was so fearful of contracting smallpox she paid an English doctor the immense sum of £10,000, plus a lifetime annuity of £500, to inoculate her and members of the imperial court. But the procedure was not always successful, and many developed severe disease and died from the rather primitive technique.

Almost fifty years later, Edward Jenner, a local country doctor in a small farming community in western England, observed during a 1788 smallpox epidemic that those who worked with cattle were somehow spared the worst ravages of the disease. There had long been rumours in rural communities that milkmaids, who were often afflicted with a much milder disease known as cowpox, were spared from the more deadly smallpox. Jenner wondered if inoculating people with cowpox could protect them from smallpox.

In 1796 Jenner was given the chance to prove his theory, when a young milkmaid named Sarah Nelmes came to him with sores on her hands, a classic symptom of cowpox. He extracted liquid from the sores and then convinced a neighbour to allow him to inject his eight-year-old son, James Phipps, with the substance. It is a measure of the fear that smallpox engendered that the farmer agreed to such a risky venture. Jenner made two small cuts in James's arm and injected him with the liquid from Sarah's sores. A few days later James came down with a mild case of cowpox but soon recovered. Six weeks later Jenner repeated the procedure on the boy, but this time he injected him with liquid from a mild case of smallpox. To everyone's relief James remained healthy — he was protected from the disease.

Jenner called this procedure "vaccination" after the Latin word *vacca* (cow). He quickly documented the successful experiment and presented his paper to the Royal Society, the most august academy of sciences in England. His theories were met with much skepticism: his learned city colleagues couldn't believe that such an important discovery had been made by a mere country doctor. Satirical cartoons depicting people sprouting cow appendages after being vaccinated appeared in the London newspapers, and Jenner was ridiculed by high society. But he persisted, even writing a book describing the many successful vaccinations he had performed and how the procedure worked. By the 1800s vaccination was in general use, and Parliament had awarded Jenner the grand sum of £150,000 to continue his work.

By the 1950s smallpox had largely been eliminated from North America, Europe, and much of South America because of the widespread use of vaccination. But in other parts of the world where vaccine was not as readily available, smallpox still took two million lives every year. In 1967 the WHO undertook the monumental task of ridding the world of the scourge forever. The campaign took more than ten years to complete, cost $300 million, and involved hundreds of thousands of health workers. They provided the vaccine to millions, from the northern reaches of the Soviet Union and China to the southern tips of South America and Africa.

Finally the greatest public health achievement against infectious disease became a reality. The last known case of the more severe form of smallpox (caused by the virus *Variola major*) was in a young Bangladeshi girl named Rahima Banu in 1975. Two years later the last natural case of the milder form of the disease (*Variola minor*) occurred in a Somalian hospital worker named Ali Maow Maalin. After three thousand years of smallpox's dominance over humankind, the WHO announced victory, declaring: "The world and all its peoples have won freedom from smallpox, which was a most devastating disease sweeping in epidemic form through many countries since earliest times, leaving death, blindness, and disfigurement in its wake and which only a decade ago was rampant in Africa, Asia, and South America."

But the cagey bug had not yet been defeated. In 1978 smallpox was accidentally released in a lab in Birmingham, England, by a virologist who was using the virus illegally in experiments. Janet Parker, a medical photographer working on the floor above, was infected with the disease and later died. Her mother was also infected but managed to survive. This senior VP of Microbes Inc. was indirectly responsible for one more victim, when the virologist who had accidentally let loose the virus committed suicide soon after.

Following this incident, smallpox specimens in laboratory samples the world over were systematically destroyed, until only two known samples remained: one at the U.S. Centers for Disease Control and Prevention in Atlanta, Georgia, and the other at the State Research Center of Virology and Biotechnology (also known as the Vector Institute) in Koltsovo, Russia. The latter sample had been moved from its home at the Institute for Viral Preparations in Moscow, following the collapse of the Soviet Union. These last known samples were scheduled to be destroyed on December 30, 1993, but they won a reprieve so scientists could debate whether the virus ought to be kept for research in case of bioterrorism attacks. Others felt the samples should be destroyed to avoid further accidents. The bug is still on death row; a second appeal was won in 1999 and a third in 2002, amidst growing concerns that some virus samples may have ended up in the hands of terrorists as the Soviet Union disintegrated. Scientists in the West are concerned that they may some day need the final samples to develop a new vaccine if the bug is released again by a rogue state.

*The Legacy of Louis Pasteur*
Vaccination remained an important technique for preventing illness, and it was further advanced by an up-and-coming French scientist named Louis Pasteur. Pasteur's early research focused on the wine and silk industries in France. He discovered that microbes were the cause of both spoiled wine and dead silkworms, and his work effectively saved these two important industries. In the mid-nineteenth century he developed a process called pasteurization, which saved countless lives from a form of tuberculosis that passed to humans through cow's milk. Pasteur also brought about universal acceptance of the germ theory of disease.

Up until the early 1800s, debate about the cause of infectious illness continued to rage in the medical community. The miasma theory, that disease was generated spontaneously by bad air, continued to be a strongly held belief among many educated men. Almost 150 years after the microscope was invented, researchers such as John Snow had proved that disease was transmitted through other means, such as water. But it was not until Pasteur and German scientist Robert Koch discovered the tiny bugs that cause illnesses that the miasma theory was laid to rest.

Pasteur can be credited for discovering bacteria and some parasites; viruses were too small to be seen by microscopes of his era and would not be discovered for another sixty years. His new-found bugs formed the basis of the germ theory: micro-organisms, not bad air, cause infectious diseases. Once the germ theory was established the medical world invested its energy in finding ways to stop the bugs.

It was late in his career that Pasteur developed the vaccine that he became most famous for, one that prevented the fatal disease rabies. He first turned his attention to chicken cholera, a disease that decimated flocks of chickens but didn't affect humans. (The condition was named for the terrible stench of the rotting chicken carcasses, which was similar to the smell caused by the cholera bacteria in humans.) Pasteur made up batches of broth from infected chickens and diluted the liquid to see if a small amount would confer immunity without killing healthy fowl.

At first Pasteur's experiment did not yield success; all the chickens that were injected with the broth fell sick and rapidly died. But when he used broth that had been left in the lab fridge for a few weeks, the injected chickens didn't succumb to the disease. Pasteur realized that something had weakened the bugs that had been in storage. In order to prove his findings, he injected the same chickens with a dose of fresh broth and found they had been successfully vaccinated. He quickly produced samples of the vaccine that could be fed to flocks to prevent them from falling victim to the lethal circulating strains of the disease.

Pasteur next turned his attention to a disease that was decimating sheep and cattle. Using similar techniques, he developed a vaccine for the nasty spore-forming bug anthrax. He presented his work to the Academy of Sciences in Paris but was met, as so often happens with new ideas, with general disbelief. The Academy challenged him to prove that the vaccine worked. On May 5, 1881, in a public experiment that was covered by the national media, Pasteur injected twenty-four sheep, one goat, and six cows with his weakened culture of anthrax. On May 17 he injected the animals again with a slightly stronger dose of the vaccine, and on May 31 he injected them with the virulent bug. At the same time Pasteur injected twenty-four sheep, one goat, and six cows with the same strong form of anthrax. All the vaccinated animals survived and the untreated animals succumbed to the disease. This experiment was not only another triumph for Pasteur but a major advance for farmers raising livestock for human consumption. His work also resulted in continued population growth in Europe in the nineteenth century and beyond. A modern version of this vaccine was used in 2001 and 2002 to protect people exposed to anthrax-laced letters that terrorized parts of the United States.

Pasteur's next target was rabies, a disease that had horrified him since childhood, when he witnessed a man die a crazed and painful death after being bitten by a rabid dog. Though he didn't know it at the time, Pasteur was looking for a virus, and viruses are much more difficult to grow in a lab than bacteria. But he applied the same principles and a similar technique, using dried brain tissue from infected animals. He eventually developed a vaccine that would protect not only animals but people as well. Because there was great concern about the safety of these new vaccines, Pasteur would not test them on humans. Instead he suggested that all dogs in the country receive the vaccine as a way of controlling the disease.

Then, on July 6, 1885, a terrified woman came to Pasteur with her nine-year-old son, Joseph Meister. Joseph had been bitten repeatedly by a rabid dog, and his death was certain if he couldn't get help. Pasteur agreed to treat the boy, and injected him with fourteen doses of the rabies vaccine over the next ten days. The boy survived and Pasteur's legacy was secured. In the weeks and months following, Pasteur vaccinated several thousand others and even saved nineteen Russian peasants who had been attacked by a rabid wolf. The czar of Russia was so grateful that he sent Pasteur a hundred thousand francs, which he used to start the now world-famous Pasteur Institute in Paris. Joseph Meister would grow up to become the gatekeeper at the Pasteur Institute. In a tragic epilogue to the story, Meister committed suicide in 1940; rather than comply with Nazi demands that he open Pasteur's crypt, which was housed at the site, he took his own life.

The rabies vaccine available today is a direct descendant of Louis Pasteur's early discovery. Though Edward Jenner had invented the concept of vaccination almost a hundred years earlier, he had used a surrogate bug, cowpox, to formulate his vaccine, and not every infection has such a related milder form. Pasteur was the first scientist who was able to develop a vaccine using a weakened form of the actual bug that caused the disease. This new technique had the potential to prevent so many more infections.

**Worldwide Immunization**

The early accomplishments of these medical pioneers have led to the development of numerous vaccines and control worldwide of infectious diseases that cost countless lives and untold suffering. A vaccine for plague, still a major killer in Europe, was developed in 1897, and during the 1920s vaccines were developed for diphtheria, a respiratory disease that was a major killer of children, and tetanus. In addition, an early vaccine for protection against whooping cough and Bacille Calmette-Guérin (BCG), an immunization that prevents severe tuberculosis in young children, were developed and used worldwide. After the Second World War, major advancements in lab technology resulted in the production of a host of other vaccines, many of which are still in use today.

Vaccines and clean water systems are widely regarded as two pillars of public health that have had tremendous impact on the world's health. Today we live in a world where we no longer worry about the destruction caused by those leaders of Microbes Inc. But it took many years before this achievement could be realized. In the early 1900s vaccines were available only to those who could afford them, and widespread immunization was not common practice in industrialized countries until the 1970s. Rabies is almost unknown in North America and Europe, but it still causes almost 30,000 deaths a year in areas of India and Southeast Asia where the disease is common in dogs and access to vaccine remains out of reach for so many.

Buoyed by the success of the smallpox eradication program, the WHO sought to address this discrepancy in vaccine access by establishing the Expanded Programme on Immunization, or EPI. At a time when fewer than 5 percent of children in developing countries had been vaccinated against common diseases, the EPI made a concerted effort to ensure that all children were provided with six core vaccines, to prevent severe tuberculosis, diphtheria, tetanus in newborns, whooping cough, polio, and measles. Throughout the 1980s global coverage for these six vaccines increased, with some countries having more success than others; as with many public health interventions, much depended on political will, resources, and infrastructure. Many countries partnered with UNICEF and Rotary International and were able to develop programs that are still in place today.

*Summer of Fear: The Polio Story*
One international health success story transpired in what seemed to many an unlikely area. In South America a strong partnership between Rotary Canada, a world community

program aimed at improving health, education, and infrastructure in developing nations; the Pan American Health
Organization (PAHO); and the leadership of various political
groups in many countries led to the eradication of polio from
the Americas. *Poliomyelitis* is a virus that infects the human
digestive tract and is spread mainly through contaminated
water. The majority of those who are infected with the disease,
usually children, experience mild illness or no symptoms at
all. But those carrying the virus can unknowingly pass it on to
others. In about one of every two hundred cases, the disease
spreads in the blood and attacks the nervous system, leading
to paralysis and sometimes death. Polio caused widespread
outbreaks around the world for many centuries; an ancient
Egyptian tablet dating as far back as 1350 B.C. depicts a figure
with the characteristic withered leg from paralytic polio.

The debilitating disease first gained attention in North
America during a severe outbreak in children during the summer of 1916. With the advent of improved water and sewer
systems, the first exposure to the bug, which confers immunity for life, had been delayed in infants. Researchers discovered
that the polio virus tends to cause much milder disease in the
very young but has a propensity for attacking the nervous
system in older children. By the 1950s there were 21,000
cases of paralytic polio every year in the United States and
2,000 cases across Canada. The prime age of those affected
was five to nine years old.

Paralytic polio was an epidemic disease that targeted
industrialized countries with sophisticated water and sewer
systems. Every summer the virus would spread through families and communities, crippling all segments of society
equally. Parents feared for their children, who every summer
would wonder which of their friends wouldn't survive to

return to school in the fall. Images of iron lungs, braces, and aluminum crutches haunted the country. Even the most affluent families could not escape. Perhaps polio's most illustrious victim was a man who became American president, Franklin D. Roosevelt. In Canada the then minister of health Paul Martin had been afflicted with the disease as a child, as was his son Paul Martin Jr., who survived to become a long-serving finance minister, then prime minister of Canada in 2005.

Major epidemics hit both the United States and Canada in 1931, and in 1937 the unprecedented rates of polio forced parents to keep their children indoors. Swimming pools and parks were closed and the start of the school year was delayed, but to no avail. Another epidemic swept the continent in 1947; in 1952 more than fifty thousand children in the U.S. contracted the disease; and the following year more than nine thousand children in Canada were infected with polio. Since the 1930s researchers around the world had been working towards developing a vaccination for the disease, but a workable vaccine had so far proven elusive.

It was during the most severe polio outbreak, in the summer of 1952, that Jonas Salk, an American scientist at the University of Pittsburgh, finally made a breakthrough. Salk managed to develop a "killed" vaccine, using Edward Jenner's early technique, made of the inactivated polio virus. But there was no way of manufacturing enough vaccine to immunize the millions of children at risk. Thankfully, a prestigious laboratory based in Toronto came to the rescue.

In 1914 John FitzGerald, a bacteriologist and public health doctor, established the Antitoxin Laboratories at the University of Toronto; its main objective was to produce an antitoxin for diphtheria. In 1917 the lab was expanded and renamed Connaught Laboratories after the Duke of Connaught,

Canada's wartime governor general. During the Second World War the lab is credited with producing a life-saving tetanus antitoxin and dried blood serum to treat shock in wounded troops.

In the 1950s a small but august group of scientists at the lab worked under the leadership of Robert Defries, who later became known as "Mr. Public Health" for his central role in developing public health systems in Canada. One of the scientists assigned to the polio problem was Leone Farrell, one of the few women researchers of her time. As children across the continent were falling victim to the paralyzing virus, Farrell worked towards producing enough of the inactive virus to allow for the mass immunization of children. Finally she hit upon what became known as the "Toronto technique." By gently rocking bottles filled with liquid and the active bug, enough of the virus could be produced, then "killed" for large-scale production of Salk's vaccine. The technique was exported to Salk's lab in Pittsburgh and to several other labs in the United States in order to begin the process of manufacturing enough vaccine for mass immunization of children across North America.

On April 12, 1955, the process of immunizing two million children across North America began — the largest immunization experiment in history. The public health initiative was a huge success, but the polio virus was not going down without a fight. Several weeks into the campaign, reports began to surface that some children had contracted polio soon after being vaccinated. These incidents were reported only in the United States, but public health officials in both countries were worried. What if this new vaccine was unsafe? What would happen to the hundreds of thousands of children who had already been vaccinated?

Disease trackers examined the specific cases in detail and confirmed that some children were contracting polio from the vaccine. Canadian Minister of Health Paul Martin had to make a decision. Should he stop the campaign and risk another summer of polio, or continue the program, hoping the vaccine in Canada was safe? It was a tense and frightening time for the country. In the end, Martin decided he had faith in the vaccine produced at Connaught Laboratories, and the Canadian immunization program continued. Investigators in the U.S. soon tracked the problem to one lab that, in its rush to produce the vaccine, had taken a shortcut during the development process and contaminated it with active virus. The lab was closed and the American immunization program resumed without further incident. Two million children were vaccinated, and that summer, for the first time in decades, there were no outbreaks of polio. The bug had been defeated.

Fifteen years later polio became the focus of international health programs in other parts of the Americas. Rotary Canada led the initiative to eradicate polio from the Americas, partnering with PAHO and countries in both North and South America to work towards this achievable goal. Although the basic public health infrastructure had improved and infant mortality rates had declined in Mexico and many South American countries, polio was still a tenacious bug in a part of the world that was unable to support those with physical disabilities. The concerted effort of Rotary, UNICEF, the WHO, and PAHO to remove this scourge crossed all political and class boundaries. What eventually came of the partnership was the realization that not every single child needed to be immunized to protect the entire community.

If we look back at what we've learned so far in this chapter, viruses can survive only by infecting a new host, and they die off if they don't find new cells to invade. To control a bug like polio it was necessary to find the pockets of children who were most susceptible to infection and ensure that they were vaccinated. The vaccinated children would provide a buffer for the relative few who hadn't been treated. If the bug can't find a new gut to infect, the outbreak would stop. This concept is called "herd immunity," and the practice was probably inspired by early vaccination trials of chickens and other domestic animals. Since the mid-nineteenth century, researchers have been aware that immunizing about 80 percent of a herd or a community means that the probability the bug will find a susceptible host is low enough that it will burn out and fade away — depending on how easily the infection is transmitted.

So the next step taken to eradicate polio from the Americas was to introduce national immunization days (NIDs). The goal was to reach 80 percent of children younger than fifteen years of age with the protective vaccine. (For other, more infectious bugs such as measles, the percentage needed to prevent an outbreak is considerably higher, closer to 95 percent.) The strategy worked, and by 1988 polio was no longer a threat to children in the Americas. These results encouraged the World Health Assembly to declare global eradication of polio by the year 2000 as its next goal.

But the regenerative power of the bug, coupled with the vagaries of human nature, made that goal elusive. Scientists soon discovered that the virus could be transmitted to new hosts even if the original host showed no symptoms of the disease. In addition, areas of human conflict where vaccination was forbidden by religious leaders or too dangerous to administer — especially in Pakistan, northern India, Afghanistan, and Nigeria — meant that the virus could find new hosts to invade. Still, the fight against polio has been a success: in 1988 there were more than 350,000 cases of polio worldwide, while only thirty-three cases were reported in 2018. More than eighteen million children have been spared from paralysis through polio immunization campaigns and more than 1.5 million have been saved from death.

Complicating the effort are rare occasions when immunization programs have lapsed, leaving large numbers of children susceptible to the disease. In some cases the vaccine triggered the spread of polio in the community. In countries such as Haiti, the Dominican Republic, Madagascar, and remote areas of the Philippines, where basic sewer systems have been destroyed or never existed, and conflict has led to the breakdown of public health systems, including immunization programs, polio has re-emerged and taken full advantage of these vulnerable societies.

❦

ONCE AGAIN WE are reminded that the leaders of Microbes Inc. have survived in this world for thousands of years, and they will not be easily expunged from our lives. Despite recent setbacks, the polio eradication program continues to protect millions of children around the world. The disease has been successfully abolished in North America, and we haven't seen even an imported case of polio for many years. The summers of fear have faded from memory. Other important childhood immunization programs in Western countries include vaccines for diphtheria, tetanus, pertussis (whooping cough), *Haemophilis influenzae* type B (a bug that causes meningitis, or infection of the lining of the brain), measles, mumps, and rubella, and now hepatitis B, varicella (chicken pox), meningitis, and pneumococcus. In fact, some of these diseases have become so rare in some countries that people are questioning the value of the vaccines.

Vaccines are in many ways the victims of their own success. We have the luxury of opting out of certain immunizations because sufficient herd immunity ensures the protection of children's health. Still, vaccination remains the most effective public health measure to protect people from infectious diseases. But the bugs of Microbes Inc. are always waiting for an opportunity to expand their reach, and a susceptible child is all they need to assert their destructive power once again.

| YEAR | VACCINE |
|------|---------|
| 1798 | Smallpox |
| 1885 | Rabies |
| 1897 | Plague |
| 1923 | Diphtheria |
| 1926 | Pertussis (whooping cough) |
| 1927 | BCG for tuberculosis |
| 1935 | Yellow fever |
| *Post–Second World War* | |
| 1955 | Polio (injectable) |
| 1962 | Polio (oral) |
| 1964 | Measles |
| 1967 | Mumps |
| 1970 | Rubella |
| 1981 | Hepatitis B |
| 1989 | Haemophilis influenzae type B (HIB) |
| 1995 | Hepatitis A |
| 1995 | Varicella (chicken pox) |
| 2000 | Pneumococcus |
| 2003 | Meningococcus (conjugate meningococcal C vaccine) |
| 2007 | HPV (human papilloma virus) |
| 2012 | Hepatitis E |
| 2018 | Ebola |

## THE SEARCH FOR A CURE

For more than two hundred years vaccination prevented many illnesses, but for much of that time the medical profession lamented the fact that we had no means to cure a person once a disease had taken hold. Early physicians believed in bloodletting, a procedure thought to rebalance the humours, or four chief fluids, of the body (blood, phlegm, yellow bile, and black bile), but in time it was recognized as a dangerous and ineffective practice. Once Pasteur's germ theory of disease was generally accepted, scientists began searching for something that could kill these germs even after the disease had taken hold. One of the first scientists to work towards a cure for disease was the German scientist Paul Ehrlich.

### Ehrlich and Early Chemotherapy

Paul Ehrlich was one of the founding fathers of modern immunology and a pioneer of chemotherapy. His initial work focused mainly on developing dyes that could be used to differentiate microbes. While the discovery of the microscope had allowed scientists to study these tiny bugs, researchers were still unable to tell them apart. Ehrlich worked towards developing a method of differentiation in order to classify each micro-organism and determine which bugs caused which diseases in humans. Some of the dyes Ehrlich developed are still in use today, including those used for the Gram stain, a standard test used in modern microbiology laboratories as a first step in identifying different bacterial species.

Ehrlich noticed that a compound he had developed called tryptan red seemed to cure mice of the often fatal disease trypanosomiasis or "sleeping sickness." He was sure he had found a "magic bullet," but to his dismay the compound didn't work on humans. He spent countless hours over the next decade conducting more experiments and manipulating components of these chemicals to create new ones that he hoped just might work. He was, in this regard, one of the fathers of modern chemistry.

In 1909 Ehrlich achieved his goal. One of his chemicals, which he named 606 because it was the 606th manipulation of the original tryptan red, worked on a disease even more dreaded than sleeping sickness. This new drug, which contained the chemical arsenic, could cure people who had contracted syphilis, a disease transmitted primarily through sexual contact. The disease's symptoms range from genital sores and rashes to effects on the nervous system. In Ehrlich's day syphilis affected thousands of people, from kings to soldiers to farmers and peasants, and in its advanced form could lead to disfiguring erosion of the nose and ears and sometimes even madness. A cure was greatly sought after, and Ehrlich's chemical 606 was the first sign of hope. He eventually named the new drug salvarsan and in 1910 introduced this new "chemotherapy" to the world. Unfortunately, though the drug did work to cure syphilis, it also had many side effects and could be lethal if doses were not administered properly. Along with giving rise to the term "chemotherapy," Ehrlich's new drug was also responsible for the saying "The cure is worse than the disease."

Over the next decades scientists around the world turned their attention to developing other forms of chemotherapy. As the science evolved and more compounds were developed to treat diseases, drug classification and naming systems also evolved. The term "chemotherapy" now refers almost exclusively to medications that kill cancer cells, but in Ehrlich's day it was used for anything that might cure disease. Since his discovery of arsenic-based medications, there has been a proliferation of drugs. Many of them, available over the counter at local pharmacies, work to reduce fevers, relieve pain, or stop your nose from running. While they don't cure diseases, they can play an important role in helping recover from illness. Salvarsan was the first of the medications known as antibiotics, which kill bacteria and can cure bacterial infections. More recently, drugs called antivirals have been developed that work on some viruses. Viruses have proven more elusive than bacteria, however; these drugs slow down their reproduction process, lessening the impact but not curing the disease.

**Antibiotics: Miracle Cures**

The next major achievement in our fight against the bad bugs of Microbes Inc. was discovered by French-American microbiologist René Dubois. Dubois had spent a good part of his career studying compounds in soil that he thought might digest and kill bacteria. He began working with Canadian-born bacteriologist Oswald Avery at the Rockefeller Institute in New York City to find a cure for *Streptococcus pneumoniae*, a bacterium that was causing a lethal form of pneumonia. Thanks to Paul Ehrlich's dyes, they were able to determine that the bug causing the disease had a strong cell wall that was made out of cellulose, a fibrous material. They began searching for a substance that would break down cellulose, believing — correctly, as it turned out — that this discovery would kill the bacteria and cure the infection.

Dubois recalled examining a specimen from a cranberry bog in New Jersey some years before that seemed to break down just about every substance in its wake. He sent for a sample and in 1929 isolated a compound he called "cranberry bog bacillus" or CBB, which digested the cell wall and killed the *Strep* in test tubes. He and Avery then tried their new compound on mice infected with the bacteria, and CBB cured them too.

In 1930 they published their findings in the journal *Science*. It was the first time a chemical from one bug had been used to destroy another, and their discovery was met with great excitement and worldwide acclaim. Unfortunately for Dubois and Avery, CBB was quickly overshadowed by the discovery of another, even more effective chemical called prontosil, which also cured disease but was much simpler to produce and did not have as many side effects in humans.

Prontosil was discovered by the German scientist Gerhard Domagk, who worked with the Bayer Company in 1927 (the same Bayer Company that discovered the wonder drug Aspirin) to search for a cure for the illness caused by *Streptococcus pneumoniae* — the same bacterium Dubois and Avery were researching an ocean away. In 1932 Domagk found a compound that cured mice, but to his surprise it had no effect on the bug in lab tests. Years later it was determined that this and its related drugs, a class now called sulphonamides or sulpha drugs, worked by damaging the bacteria and allowing the body's own immune system cells to then destroy them. Prontosil was the first of many in this class of drugs that became known as "antibiotics" and was the precursor of sulpha drugs still used today.

### Penicillin: The Magic Bullet

While this frenetic research was going on in both Europe and North America, the most important curative known to humankind was waiting to be discovered in the laboratory of

Alexander Fleming, a Scottish-born physician working at St. Mary's Hospital in London, England. Fleming had served in the Royal Army Medical Corps during the First World War and was horrified by the suffering and death he witnessed, particularly the infections that developed in the soldiers' wounds. During the war he developed techniques to treat the wounds with antiseptics to try to prevent the spread of infection. These experiences led him to devote much of his time to searching for ways to avert and also to cure disease.

Fleming first discovered a substance produced in the body, which he named lysozyme, that seemed to kill bacteria, but only bacteria that didn't cause disease. Then, in 1928, he made a more important — and serendipitous — discovery. Not a man of meticulous habits, Fleming had left some *Staphylococcus* culture plates sitting on a bench for several weeks. When he finally went to dispose of them he noticed that a fuzzy greenish-blue substance had grown on one of the plates, which he immediately recognized as a common mould called *Penicillium*. He also noticed that a protective ring had formed around the mould, leading him to conclude that something in the mould was killing the *Staph*.

Fleming managed to isolate this "mould juice" and tested the substance on *Staphylococcus* samples, as well as on a number of other disease-causing bugs, including those that caused gas gangrene and syphilis. This mould juice, which he later named penicillin, truly was the magic bullet that Ehrlich had been seeking. Penicillin was able to kill many virulent bugs without causing damage to humans. The drug rapidly replaced the dangerous salvarsan as the treatment of choice for syphilis. But it did have a downside: the substance was unstable and difficult to isolate, and when it was successfully extracted, it rapidly lost its microbe-killing properties. Fleming wasn't able to solve these problems, so he put aside his work on penicillin and moved on to other research.

Ten years later two Oxford-based scientists, Australian pathologist Howard Florey and German-born biochemist Ernst Chain, came across Fleming's paper on penicillin and began searching for ways to extract the mould juice. They developed a freeze-drying process called lyophilisation that allowed them to purify penicillin in a much more potent form and keep it stable for longer periods of time. They published their findings in 1940 after successfully testing this effective new drug on infected mice.

In 1941 Charles Fletcher, a physician at the Radcliffe Infirmary in Oxford, contacted the two men after hearing about the new drug from a colleague who worked at the pharmacy (who also happened to be Florey's wife, Ethyl). Fletcher had a patient, Constable Albert Alexander, who had developed a severe infection after scratching his cheek on a rose thorn in December 1940. It had become severely infected and Constable Alexander was on his deathbed in the Radcliffe Infirmary. Penicillin might be his only chance of survival.

Florey and Chain had tested the drug only on mice, and they were concerned about possible side effects in humans. But they were also aware that the patient would undoubtedly succumb to the infection without this new treatment. On February 12, 1941, Alexander was given an intravenous infusion of 200 milligrams of penicillin. Within twenty-four hours the patient's temperature had dropped, his appetite had returned, and the infection had begun to heal. However, because of the drug's instability and the wartime restrictions placed on Florey's laboratory, only a small quantity of penicillin had been extracted. They even took the extreme measure of distilling any remaining penicillin from Alexander's urine, but by the fifth day the medication had run out. The bacteria came back and, sadly, Constable Alexander succumbed to the infection on March 15, 1941.

Though the patient died, the experiment was without doubt a success: penicillin could cure disease. Florey and Chain channelled their efforts into finding a company that could produce the large amounts of the new drug needed to treat people effectively. The Peoria laboratory in the United States agreed to work with the scientists, and over the next three years they developed a process that enabled the mass production of penicillin. By D-Day, in 1944, the company had produced 2.3 million doses of the medication, enough to treat all the bacterial infections in the Allied troops. In 1945 Fleming, Chain, and Florey received the Nobel Prize in medicine for the discovery of this "wonder drug."

## THE USE AND ABUSE OF ANTIBIOTICS

The birth of chemotherapy in 1910 laid the groundwork for the discovery of about two hundred antibiotic compounds available today and the explosive production of antibiotics following the Second World War. These wonder drugs have saved countless lives from diseases that have plagued humans for thousands of years. By the 1960s scarlet fever was almost unknown and people were able to fully recover from wound infections, pneumonia, skin infections, and rheumatic fever; even syphilis and gonorrhea could be cured. Penicillin, the sulphas, and a third powerful antibiotic called streptomycin, which cured tuberculosis, were widely available around the world. These three medications helped advance the production of other, more powerful drugs that worked on many different classes of bacteria.

In 1959 the Surgeon General of the United States announced, "The war on infectious disease is over." Those in the medical community felt there was no longer a career to be had in investigating microbes and working on new antibiotics. Young medical professionals were told they should focus their efforts on the rising chronic conditions, such as heart disease and cancers. But the leaders of the bacterial division of Microbes Inc. would not be defeated so easily.

Almost as soon as penicillin was developed the bacteria began to change, and change rapidly, to resist the medication's killing power. After only two years of widespread use, the first penicillin-resistant bugs emerged. Today almost all strains of *Streptococcus* and *Staphylococcus*, the most common cause of skin infections, are resistant to penicillin. There may be two hundred different antibiotics on the market today, but they work in only a few different ways to kill bacteria. It didn't take long for these ever-changing and adaptable bugs to find their way around these mechanisms and to thrive again. But their efforts were also aided by human excess and error.

The widespread use of antibiotics to treat viral infections has reinvigorated the bacteria's struggle for supremacy over human populations. As we learned in our travels through the halls of Microbes Inc. most coughs, colds, sore throats, and ear infections are caused by viruses. But viruses are very different bugs from bacteria. Antibiotics were designed to work against specific proteins and components of bacteria that viruses simply don't have. Antibiotics do not cure infections caused by viruses, but our demand for antibiotics to treat these infections, coupled with doctors' reluctance to resist these entreaties, have led to widespread abuse of these medications. By taking unnecessary medications, people have provided the bacteria in their bodies with a golden opportunity to determine the way the antibiotic works, thereby exerting selective pressure on bugs that can resist the drug.

Of the millions of bugs living on our skin, only a few hundred may have the mutation that allows them to resist an antibiotic such as penicillin. If we kill off all the susceptible bugs by using penicillin for an infection caused by a virus, not only is the virus blissfully unaffected but the few bacteria with the resistant gene are given a reproductive advantage and are able to take over as the main bug on our skin. So the next time a scrape or a paper cut is infected by the bacteria on our skin, the penicillin we take to cure the infection will no longer work because the bugs are immune to the antibiotic's killing action.

In many parts of the world antibiotics are available widely and cheaply at pharmacies. In these areas the drugs are often used for any signs of infection, and not for their full course. Some people even take the medication because they believe they may prevent illness. Since the 1970s the extensive use of antibiotics that work on a number of different bacteria in animals raised for human consumption has also proven to be of great concern. Much of the food industry uses these drugs to promote growth in the animals, despite the absence of infection in a herd or flock. The long-term implications of this practice are not entirely clear, but we have seen the emergence of highly resistant bacteria in cattle, poultry, and eggs, some of which have caused outbreaks of serious illness in people. It is the emergence of these drug-resistant strains on our bodies and in our food supply that has public health officials concerned that we may run out of medications altogether that can treat infections.

## THE RISE OF THE SUPERBUG

Because of the rampant abuse and misuse of antibiotics over the past forty years, the world is now being confronted with an emerging division of Microbes Inc. that has proven to be resistant to multiple antibiotics. These multi-drug-resistant bugs have often been labelled "superbugs," not because they are transmitted more easily or even because they cause more severe disease, but because they are so much more difficult to treat than their non-resistant colleagues. The superbug that is of most concern to public health officials today is a bacteria called methicillin-resistant *Staph aureus*, or MRSA.

As we learned while touring the Bacteria Division of Microbes Inc., *Staphylococcus* is a major cause of skin and soft tissue infections, abscesses, and more rarely severe pneumonias or fatal blood infections. *Staph* is also a common cause of wound infections after surgery. Patients in hospitals are commonly on multiple- or broad-spectrum antibiotics, but because their immune systems have been compromised, they are often ill equipped to fight off infections that may result from treatment or a surgical procedure. The weakened body is the perfect environment for bacteria to develop resistance to antibiotic treatment. By the early 1990s hospitals across the United States, much of Europe, and to a lesser extent in Canada, began reporting *Staph* infections that were resistant to every drug available, with one very expensive exception: an intravenous medication called vancomycin. Methicillin resistance is a marker for this bug's ability to deflect the killing powers of many antibiotics, so these microbes became known as methicillin-resistant *Staph aureus*. These superbugs continue to cause serious complications in patients in health-care facilities around the globe.

Even more frightening is the recent emergence of a strain of *Staph* that has proven resistant to vancomycin. In May 1996 a baby in Japan developed a skin infection that defied medical treatment; even vancomycin didn't work, and the child died. This incident reminds us that we must use antibiotics wisely, or before long we may find ourselves back to the days when even a scratch from a rose thorn can be deadly. Bacteria have dominated our planet for millions of years and are experts at the game of survival of the fittest. Our belief in the potency of magic bullets has been shown repeatedly to be both naïve and deadly.

## THE PREVENTION GOSPEL

Given our limitations in preventing and treating many infectious diseases — and the misuse of the few medications we do have in our armamentarium — one cannot help but wonder how humans survive this microbe-dominated world at all. The answer can be found in the work of two other great medical thinkers whose achievements are still with us today.

### The Hygiene Story

In the 1840s, Austro-Hungarian obstetrician Ignaz Semmelweis made a critical discovery at the Vienna General Hospital. He worked there on the obstetrics ward and also performed autopsies on women who had died in childbirth of puerperal fever, or as it was more commonly known then, childbed fever. Puerperal fever was an infection of the uterus that we now know was mostly caused by the bacteria *Staphylococcus* and *Streptococcus*. But at the time Pasteur's germ theory had not yet caught on, and it was widely believed that these women died from some form of miasma, or "bad air." Semmelweis suspected that the cause of this infection was something beyond "bad air," and he made it his mission to prove his theory true.

Maternity patients were admitted to one of two wards on alternating days. Ward A was run by obstetricians and medical students and Ward B was run by midwives. Semmelweis noticed that a greater number of women were suffering from childbed fever on the ward run by the doctors; in one year he counted more than six hundred women who died after delivery on Ward A and only sixty deaths caused by the same disease on Ward B. He observed that the medical students and doctors on Ward A frequently went to the delivery ward directly after completing autopsies on women who had died from puerperal fever; midwives, on the other hand, did not perform autopsies. Semmelweis was certain that the doctors carried with them what he called "cadaver particles" from the "death rooms" and transferred these particles from their hands to new mothers during delivery. He instituted a policy that required doctors to wash their hands thoroughly in chlorinated water before they proceeded to the delivery ward.

This regulation elicited scorn and derision from the established doctors at the hospital (who likely could not bear to admit that they were responsible for the deaths of hundreds of women). But the results of the intervention supported Semmelweis's theory: within one year the mortality rate among maternity patients had decreased substantially. In 1847 the monthly death rate from childbed fever on Ward A was as high as 18.3 percent. In the year after Semmelweis enforced the handwashing regulation, the rate fell to as low as 1.2 percent, and for several months no deaths were reported at all. Semmelweis received support for his initiative from a number of young and more progressive doctors, but the establishment was resistant to change and eventually won the day. The handwashing requirement was abolished and death rates on Ward A rose again, to higher levels than ever.

Semmelweis was a difficult and bitter man, and in his later years he developed severe psychosis and was eventually admitted to an asylum. Ironically, he died from an infected wound in 1865, at only forty-seven. It was not until much later that Semmelweis's handwashing edict was recognized among health officials throughout the world as the important safety measure it is today. With the emergence of antibiotic-resistant bugs, the importance of what we now call "hand hygiene," which includes both handwashing and the use of alcohol-based hand rubs, has made an impressive resurgence in health-care facilities around the globe. Studies in recent years have shown that health-care workers wash their hands only 40 to 60 percent of the times they should while caring for patients. These figures are alarming, considering that we now know that infections are too often transmitted by direct contact. Microbes are ever-present, even though we can't see them with the naked eye, and all bugs — even superbugs — are not immune to handwashing.

## Joseph Lister and Hospital Hygiene

The second person who contributed much to our present-day understanding of the transmission of disease was Joseph Lister, an English surgeon who was working at the Glasgow Royal Infirmary in the mid-1860s. Like Semmelweis, Lister was also concerned about the number of fatal infections that occurred in patients after surgery. Even if the surgery was a success, far too many patients died afterwards from rotting infections in their wounds. English nurse and medical reformer Florence Nightingale had started a crusade to clean up and air out hospital wards to help reduce mortality rates in patients recovering from treatment. But her ideas were not well regarded, and most surgeons still clung to the belief that infections were a result of a nasty miasma.

Lister found out about Pasteur's germ theory after reading a paper Pasteur had published on fermentation. Lister was convinced that there was something he and his colleagues were doing that caused some of these infections. He instituted a hygiene policy, which required all surgeons to wash their hands, disinfect their instruments in carbolic acid (phenol) before surgery, and clean wounds with a dilute solution of carbolic acid. He also required surgeons to wear clean gloves for each procedure and to spray the air with carbolic acid, which was used at the time to reduce the stench of rotting sewage and was thought to have some microbe-killing properties.

These measures dramatically reduced the rates of infection at the Glasgow Royal Infirmary, and Lister wrote up the results of his policy in a seminal paper called "Antiseptic Principles of the Practice of Surgery," which was published on September 21, 1867, in the prestigious medical journal *The Lancet*. Unlike poor Semmelweis, Lister and his ideas were embraced immediately by the medical community, and he became a well-respected and sought-after surgeon. He continued his work developing improved means of antisepsis, and in 1879 the mouthwash Listerine was named after him. He retired in 1893 but was still called upon to advise upon important matters; he even oversaw an operation on King Edward VII, who had developed appendicitis two days before his coronation in 1902. The king recognized the importance of the disinfection measures Lister implemented and acknowledged he likely would not have survived had it not been for Lister's work. His comment is in no way an overstatement; surgery for appendicitis was still a rare and often deadly procedure in those days.

By ensuring that surgical instruments were disinfected and the hands of hospital staff were always clean, Lister revolutionized the way we think about infectious disease. A century and a half later his preventive measures continue to be practised in hospitals throughout the world.

❀

IN OUR MODERN world of crowded cities and overburdened hospitals, where misuse and abuse of antibiotics are common and some fear vaccinations, the work of Semmelweis and Lister reminds us that prevention is key. The most important and effective measure we have to prevent getting sick is to wash our hands. The players of Microbes Inc. are indeed formidable foes. In the next chapters we will resume our tour of this global corporation, taking a closer look at bugs that transmit disease through the air and through our food and water, and those that we confront on our travels, and even in our own backyard.

# BUGS IN OUR WORLD

# THREE

## BUGS IN
## THE AIR

O N MARCH 8, 2003, a forty-four-year-old man sat in the emergency department of a busy community hospital in Toronto, Ontario. He was coughing and feverish. His sister sat with him for a few hours but then had to leave to look after their mother's funeral. Their mother had died just three days before; the coroner had concluded that the cause of death was a heart attack brought on by the severe viral infection she had been suffering from a few days before her passing. She had just returned from a visit to her native Hong Kong and surely had picked up the bug there. That and the long trip had worn her out.

The young man had started feeling unwell about a day before his mother died. He lived in the same house as his parents, along with his wife, their young son, and his brother. Now he would miss the funeral while he lay on a stretcher in the crowded emergency ward. There were no beds available in the hospital, so he spent the night coughing into his oxygen mask in the small observation area he shared with six others. Little did they know that SARS, the biggest and most frightening outbreak in Canada since the 1918 influenza pandemic, had been unwittingly unleashed upon the City of Toronto.

✣

MANY VIRUSES AND bacteria can be transmitted through the air, but the ones we encounter most often are the group known as respiratory viruses. These highly contagious bugs attach to the cells lining the upper respiratory tract, which includes the mouth, nasal passages, throat, and upper airways of our lungs. Once they have invaded these outer protective cells they cause what we in the medical community call "upper respiratory tract infections" or URIs. This group of infections includes the common cold, ear infections (otitis media), sinusitis, rhinitis, and bronchitis. Almost all coughs, sneezes, runny noses, earaches, and sore throats are caused by this tenacious group of viruses.

The most common URIs are caused by a variety of rhinoviruses and adenoviruses. These small RNA viruses can mutate rapidly in order to evade the defences of our immune systems. This is why adults can catch two or three colds a year and children commonly experience up to a dozen colds or URIs annually. Let's consider some of these infections in more detail and look at the measures we can take to prevent them.

## THE COMMON COLD

The common cold has been around as long as humans have recorded history, and we are as far from a cure now as we were back in ancient times. The common cold, or acute viral nasopharyngitis, is a pesky combination of sore throat, runny nose, nasal congestion, sneezing, and coughing that lasts about a week in most people, although some symptoms can linger for two weeks or more. These ever-changing viruses are highly contagious, and spread through the air when someone coughs or sneezes. We can also inadvertently inoculate ourselves by touching our eyes or mouth with contaminated hands. For most of us a cold is little more than an annoyance, but the infection can be more severe in infants and young children when it can be accompanied by a fever and rash. And its impact on society is startling, to say the least.

Over the centuries many medical researchers have devoted their time to investigating the common cold with hopes of finding a cure. In the eighteenth century scientist, inventor, and founding father of the United States of America Benjamin Franklin set his sights on this ubiquitous illness. Even though viruses would not be discovered for another 150 years, Franklin was convinced that the common cold was somehow transmitted through the air. He observed that "people often catch cold from one another when shut up together in small close rooms, coaches, etc., and when sitting near and conversing so as to breathe in each other's transpiration." His recommendation for prevention and cure: exercise, bathing, and moderation in consumption of food and drink.

In the postwar England of 1946, the U.K. Medical Research Council set up a Common Cold Research Unit. By the 1950s researchers at the unit had discovered that the cause of the disease was a bug they called rhinovirus. Despite years of intense research, they were never able to find a cure. They did, however, do some promising work on zinc gluconate lozenges, medicinal tablets that have some benefit in preventing and treating rhinovirus infections only. The unit was closed down in 1989.

In the 1960s the Common Cold Centre at Cardiff University attempted to answer the age-old question: Does cold cause colds? They subjected volunteers to acute chilling of the feet for several hours, then monitored them for the next week to see if they developed cold symptoms. Interestingly, while the subjects of the study reported some cold symptoms, testing showed that they were not in fact infected with any of the cold viruses. Other studies since have shown no higher rates of infection in people who are chilled.

The American chemist and double Nobel Laureate Linus Pauling was also interested in finding a cure for the common cold. He was convinced that high doses of vitamin C were the remedy, and he wrote a book in 1970 called *Vitamin C and the Common Cold*, which outlined this theory. Unfortunately his results were never replicated in further studies, and vitamin C has since fallen out of favour as a cure. It is a testament to Pauling's influence that vitamin C is still widely believed to prevent or treat colds, though it is no longer taken in the large doses he espoused.

We now know that the common cold is caused by more than ten different types of rhinovirus as well as a variety of other viruses, including coronaviruses, adenoviruses, parainfluenza virus, respiratory syncitial virus, and some enteroviruses. With more than a hundred respiratory viruses causing colds, it is no wonder that a cure is elusive. In the United States alone a hundred million people a year visit a doctor to receive treatment for the common cold. As a result, more than 150 million workdays are lost and as many as 180 million school days are missed at a cost of somewhere around $20 billion every year.

In addition to the economic impact, as many as a third of patients are prescribed antibiotics, which are medications developed to fight bacterial, not viral infections. These prescriptions have led to over $1.1 billion in unnecessary costs and, more ominously, to the development of antibiotic-resistant strains of bacteria. Americans also spend in the vicinity of $3 billion a year on over-the-counter medications and $400 million on prescription medications, all for symptomatic relief of the common cold.

We have tried everything from vitamin C to echinacea to zinc to lemon tea, not to mention pharmaceuticals such as decongestants, cough suppressants, antihistamines, and anti-inflammatories. Recent studies have shown that these medications have little benefit and can be downright dangerous for young children; the infant versions of these medications have been removed altogether from pharmacy shelves. In the end, the only certain cure we have for the common cold is time. Far better, then, to prevent catching a cold in the first place.

The single most important and effective measure we can take to prevent transmitting those pesky cold viruses is to wash our hands. Washing your hands with warm water and soap or cleaning them with an alcohol-based hand sanitizer at least five times every day reduces the risk of catching the common cold or spreading infection to others. Antibiotics are not going to help and may cause more harm in the long run. And remember that old saying, "Feed a cold and starve a fever"? While there is no scientific evidence to back it up — at least not the starving bit — I personally would never underestimate the healing power of chicken soup to provide comfort and relieve suffering.

## INFLUENZA

Another respiratory virus that routinely causes serious illness is influenza or, more correctly, the family of influenza viruses. There are three types that we need to be concerned about: influenza A, B, and C. Of these the most serious by far is influenza A, which has been known to cause worldwide pandemics. This highly contagious disease likely originated in wild aquatic birds such as ducks or geese, but it can also be found in pigs and, less commonly, dogs, horses, camels, ferrets, cats, seals, mink, whales, and no doubt other species that have not yet been tested. Influenza B, on the other hand, affects mostly humans, and the only other species shown to have contracted the infection is, somewhat surprisingly, seals. Influenza C viruses rarely cause disease in humans (occasionally they affect pigs); its symptoms are similar to those of the common cold. It is influenza A's unique ability to spread to a vast array of species that makes it especially dangerous to humans.

Influenza, or "the flu," is a particularly nasty combination of fever, chills, cough, shortness of breath, muscle aches, weakness, and headaches. In young children this viral infection can also cause nausea and vomiting; it is sometimes confused with "stomach flu," or gastroenteritis, which is caused by other viruses that attack the gut. "The flu" really refers to the respiratory disease caused specifically by the influenza viruses, and its symptoms tend to be much more severe than those caused by the common cold or the many troublesome stomach bugs. In young children, the elderly, and anyone whose immune system is weak or has been compromised, influenza can lead to more serious infections such as sinusitis, bronchitis, ear infections, and even pneumonia.

Influenza A was first described by the Greek physician Hippocrates more than 2,400 years ago. The first detailed record of an outbreak was made in 1580 and describes the spread of the disease from Asia through Africa to Europe. In Rome more than eight thousand people perished, and in several Spanish cities populations were wiped out entirely by this devastating disease. Throughout the seventeenth, eighteenth, and nineteenth centuries influenza epidemics continued to decimate populations, and during the 1900s there were three major worldwide outbreaks or pandemics. The most notorious was the Spanish flu of 1918–19, which killed an estimated forty million people around the world. In 1957 the Asian flu killed as many as two million people, and in 1968 the Hong Kong flu was responsible for one million deaths.

Today influenza continues to have a devastating effect on populations throughout the world. This is because every year the influenza viruses change enough to evade our immune systems and cause sickness and death. Annual or seasonal influenza generally peaks in the winter, which in the northern hemisphere is from October to March and in the southern hemisphere from June to September. The WHO estimates that 5 to 15 percent of the world's population is affected by influenza every year, with three to five million severe cases requiring immediate medical attention or hospitalization and 250,000 to 650,000 cases resulting in death. In the developed world most of the hospitalizations and deaths occur in the elderly and chronically ill, those whose immune systems are unable to fight off the virus.

We know much less about influenza's impact on the developing world, but we do know that the viruses cause illness year-round in many tropical regions. We also know that influenza's attack rates and mortality rates in developing countries have been shockingly high. One such outbreak in Madagascar in 2002 caused severe illness in twenty-seven thousand people, and eight hundred died in just under three months, despite rapid intervention. This is just one example of the devastating effect of influenza on a vulnerable population with limited access to health care. The numbers are staggering, and they have triggered a great deal of public health research in the past twenty-five years to try to reduce both the annual impact of influenza outbreaks and the potential impact of the next pandemic.

Influenza was first discovered in 1931 by the American pathologist and virologist Richard Shope, who found the virus in pigs. Shortly thereafter, in 1933, British scientist Patrick Laidlaw from the Medical Research Council in the U.K. was the first to isolate the virus in humans. By 1944 the first influenza vaccine had been developed at the University of Michigan by Thomas Francis Jr., an American physician, virologist, and epidemiologist. Much of his research was funded by the U.S. Army, which was anxious to develop a vaccine for a disease that had caused unparalleled damage to the military during the Spanish flu pandemic at the end of the First World War.

Influenza viruses have been described by researchers at the WHO as "promiscuous, sloppy, and capricious." They are considered "promiscuous" because their RNA is broken into eight small pieces instead of being one long strand, which allows these viruses to trade bits of genetic material with each other. The gene swapping, or reassortment, gives birth to a new, hybrid influenza virus that can evade the immune system's defences. This process is known as a "genetic shift," and as we say in the business, "shift happens." When it does happen, pandemics can follow.

Influenza viruses are labelled "sloppy" because having only a single strand of genetic material (RNA) means they can replicate rapidly and without the hindrance of a double-checking mechanism. So when they do replicate, errors, or small mutations, are common. These frequent small errors in the virus's genes means that it will "drift," or change a bit, every year, which explains why a new vaccine must be developed every year to combat the latest circulating strains of influenza.

Finally, these "capricious" viruses can slow down their replication process in order to adapt to their new environment. This process, called adaptive mutation, allows a virus to acclimatize to its human host and then spread easily and rapidly to other human hosts. All in all, this unpredictable bug has evolved — and continues to evolve — rapidly, to the consternation of scientists and public health officials the world over. It truly is a moving target.

In order to obtain some understanding of the changing virus and what strains are causing illness in people, the WHO established the Global Influenza Surveillance and Response System, with 152 national influenza centres in 113 countries. Each laboratory monitors the strains of influenza circulating in its area of the globe, checking for drifts and for the more worrisome and potentially deadly shifts. Twice a year scientists from the network hold a meeting to determine which viral strains will make up the next season's influenza vaccines, one for the northern hemisphere and one for the southern hemisphere.

One of the key pieces of data that the Global Influenza Surveillance and Response System has uncovered are two proteins coded in the eight genes of the influenza A virus. These viruses have two surface proteins: the H protein, or hemagglutinin, which allows the virus to bind to blood cells, and the N protein, or neuraminidase, which allows the release of progeny virus from the infected cell. There are limited known combinations of these proteins, and to a large extent they determine whether the virus will be effective and efficient in infecting people. So far we know there are sixteen H types (H1–16) and nine N types (N1–9); all of the possible H and N combinations are found in aquatic birds, but only a few are known to cause infections in humans.

Scientists have adopted a somewhat complex naming system to be able to tell if the same, slightly different, or entirely new strains of influenza A are spreading among populations. The circulating influenza A viruses are named for their H and N type, as well as for where they originated and in what year. Since 1977 we have seen two slightly different strains of influenza A — influenza A/Wisconsin/67/2005 (H3N2) and influenza A/Brisbane/59/2007 (H1N1) — and one strain of influenza B, influenza B/Florida/4/2006. The H3N2 strain was composed of a virus with H3 and N2 proteins, was first found in Wisconsin in 2005, and was the sixty-seventh strain seen that year. A cousin of the H3N2 virus that has the genes for the H1 and N1 proteins was first detected in Brisbane, Australia, in 2007, and was the fifty-ninth strain detected that year.

Influenza B viruses don't change as rapidly and descend primarily from two main lines, Victoria and Yamagata. The viruses were named after the areas in which they were first detected: Victoria, Australia, and Yamagata, Japan. The Florida strain found in 2006 was a slight drift along the Yamagata line. While the coding system may seem complex, it provides a clear common language for scientists worldwide, allowing them to exchange valuable information about potential new strains from around the globe.

## The Rise of Bird Flu

So far, only influenza A strains with H1, H2, and H3 proteins are known to cause epidemic disease in people. But viruses with all the H and N protein types can cause disease in domestic poultry, and on a few occasions these infections have spilled over to humans. In 2003 four people developed eye infections after being exposed to an outbreak of influenza H7N7 on chicken farms in British Columbia, and an outbreak of H9N2 in poultry in the Netherlands that same year caused mild infections in several people and resulted in one death, a veterinarian who had visited an affected barn.

The process of breeding poultry in high-density environments to produce more meat has led to the loss of the genetic diversity that once protected the birds from infections. Avian influenza outbreaks now happen with greater frequency in poultry operations because of this industrialization. Some of these viruses cause mild disease. The chickens may become lethargic and produce fewer eggs; these are called "low-pathogenic strains." Less common are the "high-pathogenic strains" of influenza A, which first cause sniffles and then roar through poultry barns, rapidly killing the captive birds. The issue that concerns the WHO and public health doctors around the world is that if one of these highly pathogenic strains can make the leap — by reassortment or mutation — to becoming effective at infecting humans, we may have the next influenza pandemic on our hands.

Our first brush with this potential disaster came in 1997, when a new strain of influenza A was discovered in poultry in the wet markets of Hong Kong. This H5N1 strain infected eighteen people, mostly children; all of them were admitted

# How Do Flu Pandemics Occur?

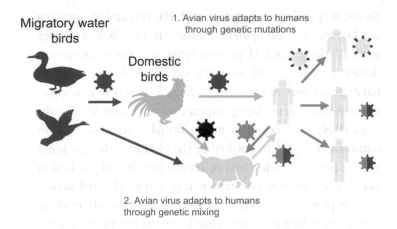

Migratory water birds

1. Avian virus adapts to humans through genetic mutations

Domestic birds

2. Avian virus adapts to humans through genetic mixing

to hospital, and six died. This incident alarmed public health officials worldwide. Not only was the mortality rate astonishingly high, but those who succumbed to the disease died of a strain of influenza thought not to affect humans. Clearly this was something new and dangerous.

The WHO worked with local authorities and in three days destroyed more than 1.5 million chickens infected by or exposed to the new virus. Their actions may have averted a pandemic, and they certainly raised the collective consciousness of health officials around the world. Since then the WHO has been developing emergency response systems for future threats and encouraging governments to plan and prepare for another potentially deadly global crisis. Some experts feel that another influenza pandemic is inevitable and that the capricious, sloppy, promiscuous influenza virus is lying in wait for the ideal circumstances to wreak havoc on populations around the world. As some have said, "The clock is ticking. We just don't know what time it is."

Adding fuel to the fire was the re-emergence in 2003 of the nasty influenza A H5N1 strain that caused such concern in Hong Kong in 1997. The virus first spread in China, and by the time public health officials became aware of the situation, the disease had spread to chickens, ducks, and geese in Vietnam, South Korea, Thailand, and Indonesia. Over the next five years this new H5N1 strain spread to poultry across Southeast Asia and to Russia, Eastern Europe, Europe, the Middle East, and some countries in Africa. So far the only areas of the globe spared from avian influenza H5N1 have been the Americas.

The first human cases of avian flu were reported in 2003 in Vietnam. By 2008 over 387 people in fifteen countries were known to have contracted this new strain of influenza, and about 60 percent died from the virus. In addition, while thankfully still rare, there have been cases of human-to-human transmission in families in Thailand and Indonesia. If this new H5N1 strain can mutate or reassort with a human strain, it may just develop the capacity to spread rapidly and efficiently among populations — and most people will have no immunity to it.

## The Fight Against Influenza

Scientists have been trying to develop a vaccine against influenza H5N1 since the disease first appeared in Hong Kong more than ten years ago. Influenza vaccines are developed by growing the virus in eggs, killing the virus, and then extracting the proteins for the vaccine. The body's immune system recognizes these proteins and develops neutralizing antibodies that protect us against infection from the virus. But the H5N1 strain has proven so deadly that even small amounts of the virus kill the eggs when injected. New techniques of growing the virus in cell lines look promising, but so far there is no effective immunization for this deadly strain.

The other tool in our armamentarium is a class of medications called neuraminidase inhibitors (NIs). First developed in the late 1990s, these drugs work by blocking the N protein and preventing the newly replicated virus from leaving the infected cell. Currently there are two NIs on the market: zanamivir (brand name Relenza®), a powder that is administered through an inhaler, and oseltamivir (brand name Tamiflu®), which comes in pill form. While NIs can't stop the spread of influenza, they can reduce the length of time patients suffer from the disease and decrease the chance of contracting secondary infections such as bacterial pneumonias.

When the new strain of influenza H5N1 emerged in 2003 in Southeast Asia, NIs were used to treat patients, but with limited success. The crisis triggered governments of developed countries to stockpile NIs (mostly oseltamivir because of its easy-to-use pill form) to safeguard against an avian flu pandemic. But supplies are limited, and there is no guarantee the medication will work.

Key members of the WHO and governments from around the world are locked in an ongoing debate about whom the medications ought to go to if a pandemic should break out and how they will be distributed. Should the medication be used to treat those who have contracted the illness or should they be given to health-care workers and other key people who will be needed to provide care? There are no easy answers to this difficult ethical question, and a lot more thought and discussion need to take place before we can determine which plan will benefit the most people.

To complicate matters further, the Global Influenza Surveillance Network discovered that the circulating strains of influenza were developing resistance to oseltamivir. In 2008 researchers in Denmark discovered a mutation in a strain of H1N1 that allowed it to resist the effects of oseltamivir. Since then scientists have uncovered this mutation in varying degrees around the world, from 10 to 15 percent of the strains in North America to 100 percent of the viruses tested in South Africa. Knowing what we do about the remarkable adaptability of the top executives of Microbes Inc., it should come as no surprise that these viruses have already found ways to foil this drug. It does, however, lead to considerable uncertainty about our ability to protect people against the next pandemic.

### Mexico and the Swine Flu

While all eyes were on the East, a new strain of influenza was quietly evolving in Mexico. On April 20, 2009, officials sent samples from fifty-one young Mexicans hospitalized with severe pneumonia to the National Microbiology Laboratory in Canada, with an urgent request to help identify the bug that was causing the illness. Doctors in Mexico City had alerted national public health authorities a few days earlier that previously healthy young people were being admitted to their hospitals with severe atypical pneumonias. Some required ventilators to help them breathe and several had died. Influenza season had come late in Mexico; cases of influenza-like illness started to rise by mid-March and then increased dramatically throughout April. Fear sprang up that this severe illness was being caused by a new and deadly bug.

Public health authorities quickly scanned other hospitals in and around Mexico City. Sure enough, doctors in the surrounding area also reported treating young people, mostly between the ages of twenty-five and forty-four, with severe respiratory illness. Mexican health authorities reported to their colleagues in Canada about two clusters of illness: one in Mexico City, where 120 people had fallen ill and thirteen had died, and another about 150 kilometres north of the city, in San Luis Potosí, where fourteen people had severe illness and four had died. The Canadian laboratory set out to find the cause of the disease and within days identified a new strain of influenza in eighteen of the original fifty-one samples that had been sent to them from Mexico. What they discovered was a triple reassortment; somehow the bug had picked up genes of avian, human, and swine origin to form a brand-new combination. Although this new virus was technically an influenza A H1N1 strain, it was not the same as the human H1N1 that had been causing illness for the past few years. This new bug quickly became known as swine flu because the major new genetic pieces originated from pigs. By the time that it was discovered, however, none of the cases in Mexico had had contact with swine before falling ill; the virus had become well adapted to transmit between people.

While Mexican and Canadian health officials were deciphering this new virus, the U.S. CDC were investigating something new of their own. They had received two flu samples from unrelated children in California that were unusual. The first was from a ten-year-old boy in San Diego County who had become ill with fever, coughing, and vomiting on March 30, 2009. He was taken to an urgent-care clinic on April 1 for assessment. A swab was taken at the clinic as part of a clinical trial to evaluate a new influenza test. The child recovered uneventfully, but he tested positive for a new type of influenza A that couldn't be identified. The local investigators sent the sample to the CDC for further evaluation.

The second sample was from a nine-year-old girl who lived in Imperial County, California. On March 28 she became ill with a cough and fever and on March 30 was taken to a clinic for treatment. The clinic was participating in a special influenza surveillance project, so a swab was taken from the girl. She was treated and recovered, but her test also showed an unusual strain of influenza A that could not be identified. It too was sent to the CDC laboratory for more detailed tests.

On April 17 the CDC announced that both specimens had been identified as a new strain of influenza A H1N1, but the virus was of swine origin, not human. Public health officials and scientists from Mexico, the United States, Canada, and the WHO collectively held their breath. Were these new strains the same, and did this mean that a new influenza virus that was causing severe disease in Mexico had already spread to the U.S.? Within days the answer came back: yes, the two strains were the same, and yes, not only were people contracting the virus in the U.S. but the infection was also widespread throughout Mexico and cases were being reported in Canada too.

The WHO raised its pandemic alert level to four and then to five after it became apparent that this new strain was causing illness in hundreds of people across North America. Although initially most who contracted the infection had travelled to Mexico, by the end of April it was clear that this influenza was being passed between people in communities across the continent. Most cases in Canada and the U.S. were relatively mild; very few people needed hospitalization and there were even fewer deaths. In Mexico a more detailed epidemiologic investigation revealed that thousands of people across the entire country were ill with this new infection; the young people with severe illness were just the tip of the iceberg. In early May the WHO reported that twenty-nine countries around the world had officially declared 3,440 confirmed cases of the swine flu and forty-eight deaths, but sustained transmission beyond travellers was still confined to North America.

It is hoped that, as the influenza season wanes in North America, this new strain will wane as well. But what will happen when influenza season ramps up again in the fall? Will this strain come back in a more virulent form and cause severe infections and deaths? A look at past pandemics shows this scenario to be a possibility. The Spanish influenza pandemic of 1918–19 made its first appearance as a relatively mild influenza that caused disease in Europe in May and June 1918. But the virus came back with a vengeance in the fall, causing the worst pandemic in recorded history and killing millions around the world. The medical community is watching closely to see what happens in the southern hemisphere in the next few months as they enter their influenza season. If the swine flu starts picking up and causing more severe illness in Australia and New Zealand, it may be a harbinger of the fall season in the northern hemisphere.

Scientists are now working to grow the virus in the lab — the first step in making a new vaccine that may be ready in time for the next flu season. But big dilemmas remain: If we put all our efforts towards a new vaccine, how will that affect our ability to produce a vaccine for the other flu strains that are still circulating and causing people to get sick and die? As well, this new swine influenza H1N1 is sensitive to the NIs (oseltamivir and zanamivir), so how should we use the stockpiles that countries have amassed? Will this new strain be the cause of the next big pandemic or will it just fade away? For now we are watching closely and making preparations for the worst-case scenario. Only time will tell.

So what can we do to protect ourselves and our families when so much is unknown? Like the common cold, influenza spreads when someone who is infected with the virus coughs or sneezes. The virus can also remain active on surfaces such as doorknobs and taps or in a drop of water or mucus for anywhere from a few minutes to several hours. Our best and perhaps only defence is what we in the medical field call "respiratory etiquette." This means covering your mouth when you cough or sneeze, preferably with a tissue that can be disposed of immediately. If you don't have a tissue, cough or sneeze into your sleeve. It sounds funny, but this technique keeps those flu bugs from flying into the air and infecting others. The next step is to wash your hands or use alcohol-based hand rubs to stop the spread by direct contact and to kill any viruses that may linger on your hands. Finally, stay at home if you have a fever. A fever is a sure sign your body is fighting off something that could be passed on to others. These three measures may be our first and perhaps only line of defence against the next influenza pandemic.

## THE SARS STORY

While the world's disease detectives were on the hunt for shifting influenza viruses, SARS emerged quietly and lethally in the rural areas of China's Guangdong Province. While public health officials' attention was turned towards the new H5N1 avian flu that was causing severe respiratory disease in people in China, researchers believe that two or more coronaviruses mutated to create a virulent new bug. Before the emergence of SARS, coronaviruses were known to cause only mild colds in people. They have since proven to be a greater cause for concern.

Guangdong Province, and in particular its capital city, Guangzhou, is known throughout China for restaurants that serve highly prized wild animal meat. People from across the country flock to the area to dine on these extravagant meals. Everything from poisonous snakes to bears to exotic animals such as the Chinese ferret badger, raccoon dog, and Himalayan masked palm civet cat is on the menu. The latter three species are often infected with coronaviruses, and one of them was likely the source of the nasty human illness we now know as SARS.

When epidemiologists traced the origin of the SARS outbreak in 2003, they found the first cases in cooks who worked in the exotic restaurants in Guangdong. They also came across densely crowded markets crammed full of caged wild animals. When SARS first appeared in November 2002, most patients were treated at a local hospital in Guangzhou. Rumours started circulating in health-care chatrooms: something new and deadly had emerged in the region. But when pressed for information by the WHO, the Chinese government would say only that there was a small outbreak of "atypical pneumonia" that they believed was caused by an unusual bacterium called *Chlamydia pneumoniae*. Early in 2003 they reported that the outbreak was over, and in the end resulted in three hundred cases and only five deaths.

Despite the government's efforts to assuage concerned citizens, the rumours persisted. Health officials in the neighbouring cities of Hong Kong and Shanghai began monitoring hospitals for cases of severe respiratory infections. The City

of Shanghai actually developed a detailed and effective surveillance program for this new infection, which probably
saved it from a more devastating outbreak of SARS. Despite
these precautionary measures, there was no way of tracking
the tens of thousands of people who travelled to and from
Hong Kong every day. The virus made its way undetected
into the territory in February 2003.

SARS began its global journey in the breathing passages of
a Guangzhou doctor who travelled to Hong Kong for a family
wedding. He had been treating patients who had contracted
this new infection and was mildly unwell when he landed in
Hong Kong. He then checked into the Metropole Hotel —
now infamous in international epidemiology circles — where
he stayed in room 911 on the ninth floor. Over the next few
days his condition worsened, and on February 22, 2003, he
was admitted to a local hospital.

Two people who had visited with the doctor on the ninth
floor were admitted to hospitals just days later, and this
unleashed the largest outbreak of SARS in Hong Kong. One
traveller who also had a room on the ninth floor returned to
Vietnam and spread the contagious disease there, while
another ninth-floor resident returned to Singapore with the
same deadly consequences. One young man flew home to
San Francisco, but thankfully the disease did not spread
there. A couple arrived in Vancouver and were promptly isolated by hospital staff after describing their recent travel and
stay at the Metropole Hotel; transmission in this case was
limited as well.

But when an elderly woman and her husband flew home
to Toronto after spending three nights on the ninth floor of
the Metropole Hotel, the woman became ill. She went to see
her family doctor, who reassured her that she had a viral

infection and counselled her to rest. Tragically, she died at home on March 5, 2003. The coroner stated that her death was due to her heart condition, which was most likely aggravated by diabetes and the viral infection she had recently contracted. What her family understood was that she had died in her bed from a heart attack.

Three days later the woman's eldest son, who lived in the same house as his mother along with his wife and young child, fell ill. He was taken to the local hospital and admitted with pneumonia on March 8. The forty-four-year-old man's illness did not raise any alarm bells at the hospital, and nobody thought to place him in isolation — he had not travelled in six years, and it was not uncommon for patients to contract respiratory infections during the winter months in Toronto.

The man was placed in an observation area with six other people until a room became available in the main ward of the hospital. Thirty-nine hours later he was transferred to the intensive care unit. The ICU doctor was worried that the patient might be suffering from tuberculosis, a disease still seen all too frequently in the multi-ethnic population that lived in the area. He put the man in an airborne-infection isolation room to protect the other patients and staff, and notified the local public health department. Unfortunately, however, SARS had already spread to at least fifteen people by that time. The largest outbreak of the disease outside Asia had been unleashed.

Officials at the public health department soon realized that several members of the man's family, including his wife, brother, sister, and even his six-month-old son, were also sick with fever and a cough. On March 13 the man succumbed to the illness, just hours after the WHO had issued its first alert about a severe new respiratory illness circulating in China and Hong Kong. Within hours of his death several family members were diagnosed with severe respiratory infections. His brother required insertion of a breathing tube; his sister and wife were sent to a different hospital. Soon after, the man's father was hospitalized as well. The only family members spared were his sister's two children and her husband. Thankfully, everyone else survived, but the catastrophic impact of SARS on their family was immeasurable.

On March 14, 2003, public health officials and local hospital staff held a joint press conference to alert the world of this dangerous new respiratory illness that was likely related to a similar disease first reported in Hong Kong. They were now in a race against time to find anyone who might have come in close contact with the family. Over the next few days it became clear that those who had shared the emergency-department observation area with the forty-four-year-old man were at great risk. An elderly patient who was being monitored overnight for chest pain had fallen ill; he was rushed to the hospital by ambulance but died the next day. His daughter and granddaughter also contracted SARS, but luckily survived. His wife, however, succumbed to the disease as well.

Before the outbreak was contained almost four months later, 375 people, mostly in the Greater Toronto Area, were infected with the disease, and forty-four had died. Among the deceased were two nurses who had bravely looked after the gravely ill, one family doctor who had treated some of the early cases, and a nurse's aide who was tending her best friend's mother. In addition, more than two thousand people who showed symptoms of the disease were examined by doctors, and more than thirty thousand were placed in quarantine — an emergency measure that hadn't been used in

Canada for almost fifty years. The negative economic impact of the outbreak cost the City of Toronto over $1 billion. Some ethnic groups, particularly Chinese communities across North America, were isolated and marginalized. Despite persistent rumours that only Asians were infected by SARS, Toronto, a truly multicultural city, proved that no one was immune to this nasty bug. By June 2003 the virus had touched every racial, religious, and ethnic group in the city.

From the outset of the crisis, public health officials and medical staff were frantically working blind. They didn't know whether the bug was a bacterium or a virus, how it was passed between people, how long it took for someone exposed to the disease to fall ill themselves (the incubation period), or whether people could pass on the disease to others before they showed signs of sickness (as happens with bugs such as measles and chicken pox viruses). They tried every resource available to them: antibiotics, which treat bacterial infections; antivirals, in case it was a virus; interferon, a drug that works against hepatitis C; and even drugs such as steroids, which counteract inflammation in the lungs. Despite these intense efforts, nothing worked. All that could be done was to support the patient's breathing by administering oxygen and to keep them as comfortable as possible to give their immune system time to regroup and fight off the bug.

Without laboratory test results, vaccines, and effective treatment, it was essential to break the chain of transmission. Those who had been in contact with the SARS virus were quarantined in their homes for ten days. If they remained in good health past the ten-day incubation period, they were released from isolation. If they began showing symptoms of the disease, they were sent immediately to hospital. There the health-care workers wore masks and other protective equipment to prevent them from picking up the virulent virus.

The one thing that became clear very early on was that the most effective preventive measure was to clean your hands. In some cases this was the only thing people could do. The City of Toronto's medical officer of health, Dr. Sheela Basrur, repeatedly reminded the public and hospital staff that the best defence against SARS was respiratory etiquette: washing your hands or using alcohol-based sanitizers, covering your mouth when you cough, and staying away from others if you felt ill. From Hong Kong to Beijing to Singapore to Toronto, this message became a worldwide mantra.

By the summer of 2003 SARS had been contained. But the outbreak exposed some serious deficiencies in our hospitals and public health systems. Hospitals in North America had been built at a time when infectious diseases were no longer thought to be a threat. They were old and crowded, and ill-equipped to detect and respond to such a massive health crisis. Infection prevention and control programs had withered because of cost-saving measures, and the public health infrastructure had been reduced to its bare bones.

The devastation of the SARS outbreak and its terrible effect on communities around the world reminded governments and the general public of the cost of losing those safety nets. Several commissions in Canada, Hong Kong, and China focused on revamping the public health system to allow for early detection of contagious disease, surge capacity to respond to new threats, and investment in hospital programs to prevent and control dangerous infections. Along with these measures came a renewed awareness of the importance of basic hygiene, especially cleaning your hands, to prevent the spread of deadly disease.

## TB THE TERRIBLE

Let's take a walk down the halls of Microbes Inc. and visit the corner office of one of the most successful players in this global corporation: tuberculosis, or TB. The bug that causes tuberculosis is a bacterium called *Mycobacterium tuberculosis*. TB can live dormant in the bodies (usually in the lungs) of people with healthy immune systems without causing illness. We call this "latent infection." The bacterium activates or begins the process of replication when the immune defences are down. Every year about one in ten people become sick this way, leading to one million new active cases of TB around the world.

About three-quarters of TB patients experience severe infection in the lungs, but TB can cause infection in almost every part of the body, including the lymph nodes, where it causes a disease known as scrofula; the bones of the spine, which leads to Pott's disease; the stomach and intestines, the pleura (the lining of the lungs), the central nervous system, and the brain. There is even a form of the disease called miliary TB, which spreads throughout the entire body. *Mycobacterium bovis*, a cousin of the TB bacterium, primarily infects cattle, but it can spread to people through the milk of infected cows. Since Louis Pasteur developed the process of pasteurization, *M. bovis* has largely disappeared.

TB is highly contagious and spreads to others when someone with active disease coughs or sneezes. It is estimated that a single sneeze from a patient with TB pneumonia can contain forty thousand droplets of aerosolized bugs. While it often takes up to eight hours of direct contact with a TB patient to become infected, on average the disease spreads to ten others before the original host seeks treatment. Throughout history TB has been given many names, from the Greek *phthisis* to the White Death to consumption, and today it affects one-third of the world population. The disease has been around for as long as man. Skeletal remains from as far back as 4000 B.C. have been found with evidence of the infection, as have mummies from 3000 to 2100 B.C. In 460 B.C. Hippocrates identified TB as the most widespread disease of his time. The Roman scholar Pliny the Elder even documented a cure for the disease, an odd concoction made up of "wolf's liver taken in thin wine, the lard of a sow that has been fed upon grass and the flesh of a she-ass taken in broth."

In 1020 the first physicians recognized that TB, or consumption, as it was known then, was highly contagious. But it wasn't until 1839 that scientists realized tuberculosis is caused by a single bacterium. This explains why over the centuries the disease has been given so many different names. In the eighteenth century its symptoms, such as red swollen eyes, pale skin, reduced temperature, and coughing up blood, were often mistaken for vampirism. By the nineteenth century TB was thought to produce feelings of euphoria — called the "hope of the consumptive"— which was believed to have facilitated creativity in the arts. Many artists and writers who became ill with TB were thought to have experienced a burst of inspiration just before death. It was also believed that the disease made women more beautiful and men more creative.

Until the late nineteenth century TB patients were treated with rest and sunshine. The first TB sanatorium was opened in 1859 in Gorbersdorf, Germany (now in Poland), by the physician Hermann Brehmer. By that time more than a quarter of all deaths in Europe were caused by tuberculosis, and most fatalities were among the urban poor. In the early 1900s the sanitation movement was involved in establishing sanatoria for TB as well as regulations to prohibit spitting in public, which was thought to be a major means of spreading the disease. In 1907 the Lung Association started the Christmas Seals campaign to fight tuberculosis, an effort that continues in modified form today.

German physician Robert Koch first identified and described the bacterium that causes TB in 1882, and in 1905 he was awarded the Nobel Prize for his discovery. That same year Albert Calmette and Camille Guérin developed the first and to date only vaccine for TB, Bacille Calmette-Guérin (BCG). It wasn't until 1921 that the vaccine was first tested on humans in France, and it was not until after the Second World War that BCG was used widely in the United Kingdom, Germany, and Canada. The vaccine was never widely used in the United States because public health officials were not convinced of its effectiveness. While BCG does offer some protection — particularly for children — against severe strains of the disease such as the miliary form, it is unable to prevent people from contracting the bug and it often complicated testing of patients for disease. Today BCG is still administered to children in areas where the number of cases runs dangerously high, but it has fallen out of use in many developed countries.

It wasn't until 1946 that scientists developed the antibiotic streptomycin, the first effective treatment for the disease. But almost as soon as streptomycin became available, the TB bug began developing resistance to the drug, and before long the bacterium was able to escape the antibiotic's killing power altogether. This is because treating TB is tricky. Not only is streptomycin a drug that is administered by injection, which must be given by a doctor or nurse, but the TB bacterium reproduces more slowly than most bacteria. Most bacteria replicate in a few minutes to a few hours, but TB, on the other hand, takes sixteen to twenty hours to reproduce and infect other cells. This means that it takes months of treatment to cure tuberculosis, while most bacterial infections are cured within a week.

In the 1950s new drugs were used in combination with streptomycin injections. The first of these was isoniazid (INH), an antibiotic in pill form, which was developed in 1952. With the advent of isoniazid, scientists thought they had finally found a cure for TB. However, most treatment regimens involved at least eighteen months of injections of streptomycin while also taking the isoniazid pills. The discovery of rifampicin (also called rifampin or RIF) in 1967 was the next big breakthrough. A combination of all three drugs meant a high probability of cure in as little as six months.

But the TB bug did not go quietly into the night. As soon as a new antibiotic was developed, the ever-changing bacterium began showing signs of resistance to the drug. In the late 1960s and early 1970s two other medications were developed: pyrazinamide and ethambutol. Current treatment for TB requires taking four drugs (isoniazid, rifampin, pyrazinamide, and ethambutol) during the first two months of treatment, then taking the two main drugs, isoniazid and rifampin, for another four months. And this is considered a short-course treatment! Despite the side effects from the antibiotics, this long and difficult treatment is our only effective means of fighting TB. All four drugs work to kill the bacterium in different ways, and because treatment and therapy run such a long course, the chances that the bug will develop resistance to all four is nearly impossible. Or so we thought.

## TB the Superbug

By the 1980s we started to see the emergence of strains of TB that were resistant to isoniazid and rifampin. This bug became known as Multi-Drug-Resistant TB or MDR-TB. Without these two key drugs, treatment for MDR-TB can take more than two years and involves medications that are many times more toxic and hundreds of times more expensive then INH and RIF. In addition, doctors are forced to treat patients with injectable drugs such as the original streptomycin.

MDR-TB now causes over 5 percent of all TB cases world-wide, and in some areas the numbers can be as high as one in five cases. Over half of the cases of MDR-TB are concentrated in China and in countries of the former Soviet Union. In Azerbaijan, for example, 30 percent of TB patients have the multi-resistant form of the bug. In September 2006, reports emerged of a strain of TB in KwaZulu Natal, South Africa, that killed fifty-two of the fifty-three people who were afflicted with the disease, and death came within days. Health-care officials discovered that this deadly strain was not only resistant to INH and RIF but to just about every other drug available to effectively treat TB. This highly lethal bug, which was named Extensively Drug-Resistant TB (XDR-TB), has now spread to 145 countries around the world, including Canada, the U.S., and many European countries. It has a frightening 90 percent mortality rate in HIV patients.

In 2007 the Centers for Disease Control and Prevention issued an unprecedented global travel alert when a young man who had been diagnosed with XDR-TB flew to Europe and back, despite warnings from public health officials. Thankfully the infection did not spread, and he eventually underwent surgery as a last-resort measure to cure the disease. But the incident reminded public health officials around the world that the spread of disease can be just a plane ride away.

❊

DESPITE ALL OF our efforts over the past fifty years, tuberculosis is still the single most successful infectious disease on our planet. In 1993 the WHO declared TB a global health emergency, and since then a program has been established to provide treatment to infected people in areas of the world where the disease is most rampant. This includes most countries in Africa as well as India, Pakistan, China, and many countries in Southeast Asia. While TB has become a distant nightmare for those who live in countries such as the United States and Canada, the devastation it still causes in countries such as South Africa, Mozambique, Russia, and China is almost unfathomable.

In 2007 the WHO estimated that there were 14.4 million active cases of TB around the world, with 9.2 million new cases in that year alone. This means that the TB bacterium infects a new person about every second! That same year 1.7 million people died from TB; the vast majority of these deaths were in Africa and Asia, where access to effective treatment is limited and many are also battling HIV and AIDS. Eighty percent of TB cases worldwide occur in just twenty-two countries.

As the SARS outbreak reminded us, no country is immune to infectious disease. In the twentieth century TB single-handedly killed more than a hundred million people. Where TB a generation ago was a widespread illness affecting every community in North America, it has now become a disease mostly of immigrants and, tragically, of aboriginal communities. Although we don't see too many cases in North America (almost 2,000 are reported in Canada each year, which works out to about five cases out of 100,000 people; it's about five per 100,000 in the United States), over 70 percent of those afflicted with TB in Canada in 2017 were immigrants from countries where TB reigns strong. Some of those countries, such as Eswanti (formerly Swaziland), have rates as high as 329 cases per 100,000 people.

Thankfully, in Canada and other Western countries treatment is available for TB and it is free for everyone. In addition, public health workers are able to prevent the disease by providing medication to those who have come in contact with a TB patient. Unfortunately many countries are unable to provide the same level of care, despite the WHO global initiative. This lack of access to hospitals and treatment facilities will allow TB to continue to thrive in many parts of the world for years to come.

## THE TALE OF DIPHTHERIA

The final stop on our tour of the respiratory division of Microbes Inc. is with a bug that was cited by *The Guinness Book of World Records* as "the most resurgent disease" on the planet. Diphtheria is an infection of the upper respiratory tract caused by the bacterium *Corynebacterium diphtheriae*. The disease was first described in the writings of Hippocrates in the fourth century B.C. and is also found in ancient Syrian and Egyptian scripts. In 1926 the French physician Pierre Bretonneau named the disease after the Greek word for leather. Diphtheria was common in France at the time, and one of its trademark symptoms is the thick, leather-like membrane that forms in the back of the throat, cutting off the airway and eventually leading to death.

During the seventeenth century diphtheria epidemics swept through Europe. The disease was known as "el garotillo" (the strangler) in Spain, and by the 1730s diphtheria had spread to North America, where it became known as "the strangling angel of children" for killing as many as 80 percent of those infected who were under the age of ten. In the 1880s the American physician Joseph O'Dwyer developed a breathing tube specifically for treating diphtheria patients. By the 1890s the German doctor Emil von Behring had developed an antitoxin serum treatment for the infection; he eventually went on to develop the first vaccine for the disease in 1913. In 1920 there were more than 200,000 cases of diphtheria in the United States with up to 15,000 deaths. Routine immunization programs were introduced that same decade, but they did not extend as far north as Alaska.

In January 1925 twenty-five children in Nome, Alaska, fell ill with the deadly bacterium. Nome at the time had a post–gold rush population of about two thousand, many of whom were native Alaskans or Inuit who had not yet been immunized against the disease. The closest treatment centre was in Anchorage, and the closest train station, Nenana, was over a thousand kilometres (674 miles) away across the bleak and frozen tundra. The local doctor put out a call to alert the authorities, and the precarious situation for those twenty-five children soon headlined news reports across the country.

A supply of the antitoxin was located in Anchorage and delivered by train to Nenana. From there, twenty-one volunteers ferried the precious antidote by dog-sled relay to Nome, using the regular mail route, the Iditarod Trail. The trip normally took on average twenty days to complete; the fastest trip ever recorded was nine days. Each volunteer team took on a leg of the trail, passing the priceless cargo on to the next team, day and night. The last leg of the journey fell to a Norwegian man named Gunnar Kaasen, whose lead dog, a black husky named Balto, forged ahead through a raging blizzard, with blinding snow and temperatures as low as minus 60 degrees Celsius.

Finally, in the early morning of February 2, the life-saving serum reached Nome. The trek had taken 127½ hours, a miraculous five and a half days. Kaasen and Balto became international heroes, and nowhere was their story better received than in New York City, where a statue of Balto still stands in Central Park. The annual Iditarod dog-sled race from Anchorage to Nome continues to commemorate this incredible journey.

Today diphtheria has been conquered in much of the world. By the late 1990s the disease had all but vanished, and from 2000 to 2007 only five cases were reported in the United States. But the bug was not about to give up. Events in some places of the world have conspired to allow its resurgence on a grand scale. Since the fall of the USSR in the early 1990s, diphtheria has re-emerged at epidemic levels in many of the former Soviet states. In 1991 two hundred cases of diptheria were reported for all of the Soviet Union; by 1998 the International Red Cross estimated that there were 200,000 cases of the disease in the same area, with 5,000 recorded deaths. In the 2000s all five cases of diphtheria in the United States were contracted by travellers returning to the former Soviet Union. When public health and immunization programs were decimated by economic and social turmoil, diphtheria had found its chance to thrive once again.

❖

THE BUGS THAT spread through the air are a varied and storied group. While we have by no means covered them all, the ones presented here are classic examples of the range and reach of respiratory bugs. They affect everyone, everywhere, and can cause unparalleled devastation. Vaccination is available for a few, but in many cases our best defence brings us back to the basics: wash your hands at least five times a day, cover your mouth when you cough, and stay away from others when you are sick. These few simple rules will keep us in good stead as we move on to the next division of Microbes Inc., the bugs that live in our food and drink.

# FOUR

# BUGS WE EAT
# AND DRINK

"BEAR MEAT BITES BACK" was the headline in a Canadian newspaper near the end of September 2005. It had been the trip of a lifetime for ten hunters from across France who set out for the wilds of northern Quebec, to hunt for bear, and it was a successful one too. The group feasted on barbecued black bear that evening in the lodge. Most had their meat prepared medium or medium rare, despite its gaminess. A few days later two of the hunters took the remains home to France to share with family and friends. Sadly, none of them foresaw the terrible impact this simple act would have only days later.

Within two weeks all ten hunters were complaining of symptoms ranging from muscle aches and headaches to high fevers, severe muscle pain, facial swelling, and inflammation of the brain. Several required extended treatment at a Paris hospital. One hunter had shared the delicacy with six relatives in central France, and half of them became ill about a week later. The other hunter shared his prize meat with seven friends soon after returning to his home in southern France, and one of the guests began suffering from the same symptoms.

All in all, fourteen of the twenty-three people who feasted on the black-bear meat contracted an illness from a parasite called *Trichinella*, a common boarder in bears, wild cats (such as cougars), foxes, dogs, wolves, seals, and walruses. *Trichinella* enters the human intestinal tract, where it releases its progeny into the blood. The larvae then migrate to the muscles, where they can live relatively protected from antibiotics for decades. Trichinellosis, the disease the parasite causes in humans, has been around for centuries, and we have known how to prevent it for almost as long — thoroughly cooking meat effectively kills the parasite. This story of international disease spread serves to remind us of the inherent risks in our food supply, and it is a small but potent example of the complexity of our global food economy.

❀

SINCE SCIENTISTS BEGAN tracking food-borne illnesses around the world, it has become painfully clear that nothing is immune to the many divisions of Microbes Inc. Common bacteria that cause food-borne illness include *Salmonella* and *Shigella*, which cause serious gastrointestinal illness, often resulting in bloody diarrhea (a sign of the severe inflammation the bug causes in the intestines), and *Escherichia coli* (E. coli), whose many strains can cause everything from mild diarrheal illness to a severe systemic disorder called hemolytic uremic syndrome (HUS), which causes bloody diarrhea and kidney damage and can be fatal.

In the Virus Division the most common bugs to cause disease through food include the Noroviruses, which bring on a short but explosive illness, symptoms of which include watery diarrhea and vomiting, and hepatitis A, a virus that affects the liver and can cause prolonged illness that may be passed on to others through contaminated food and water. In addition, several parasites have invaded our food and water systems, including *Cyclospora* and *Trichinella*, the bug that so affected the French hunters. Finally, some bacteria have the ability to produce potent toxins in humans. They go by names such as *Clostridium perfringens*, which causes the short but nasty illness that is often referred to as "food poisoning."

Food is a fundamental human need, and much of our exist-ence is spent in one way or another searching for sustenance. Since the beginning of time we have been locked in an intricate dance with the divisions of Microbes Inc. to find food that pro-vides us with the nutrition we need without giving the bad bugs direct entry into our systems, where they can make us sick. With the globalization of our food supply and the complexity of our food production systems, it has become increasingly diffi-cult to achieve and maintain this delicate balance.

In 1925 the United States Public Health Service began sys-tematically collecting and publishing information on illnesses and outbreaks related to the consumption of unpasteurized milk, and in 1938 they added information on outbreaks caused by food. The collection and analysis of this data led to the enactment of important public health standards to protect food and milk supplies. One of the first and most effective measures to be made law was the Pasteurized Milk Ordinance, which protected thousands of children from common dis-eases spread through contaminated raw milk. Meat inspection programs and animal husbandry and slaughter standards soon followed.

These programs went a long way towards protecting meat, fish, poultry, milk, and water from contamination, but over time the move to industrialized farming and large-scale food production allowed the bugs to flourish once again. Even highly processed foods are not immune to the havoc of the many divisions of Microbes Inc., and the wide geographic distribution of our food supply means that when outbreaks do occur, they can be catastrophic on a global level. Recently, for example, plants in China produced and distributed processed foods contaminated with the industrial chemical melamine, which affected people in many parts of the world. And as we will see, even the most advanced food safety and inspection programs can fail, leading to widespread illness.

In 2007 the U.S. Centers for Disease Control and Prevention estimated that more than seventy-six million Americans became ill after ingesting contaminated food, and five thousand died. In the United States alone treatment for food-borne illnesses costs the health-care system $7 billion annually. Surveillance of food- and water-borne outbreaks is a key public health function in most Western countries, including the United States, Canada, Australia, and Europe. Recently many countries have introduced sophisticated electronic tracking systems that incorporate detailed laboratory tests to allow public health investigators to trace patterns of illness in a number of locations. For example, the system can link an outbreak in Vancouver to people who have contracted the same bug from the same source in Chicago. It is hoped that making these links more rapidly will allow officials to take action sooner to prevent the spread of disease.

Some of the newer laboratory tests help identify bugs by their genetic fingerprint; the microbes can then be traced from the contaminated food to the infected people. In the past few years this system has led to the detection of *Salmonella* in almonds that were distributed across North America and to an outbreak of E. coli from prepackaged luncheon meats. Despite stringent regulations around food production and distribution, data from the surveillance system show that a whopping 6,647 food-related outbreaks were reported in the United States in 2006. This number marks a steady increase in reported outbreaks since the CDC started collecting these data in the 1930s. And this is just the tip of the iceberg: many small outbreaks aren't even reported to public health officials.

Let's take a walk through the Food and Water Department of Microbes Inc. and not only expose how global food production and distribution have led to a sharp increase in outbreaks, particularly in the Western world, but also find out what we need to do to protect ourselves and our families.

## BACTERIA

Bacteria cause some of the most severe and long-lasting illnesses related to food. In fact, over half of food- and water-borne outbreaks reported to public health officials every year are caused by this division of Microbes Inc., and the many strains of *Salmonella* are undoubtedly the disease-causing leaders.

### Salmonella

*Salmonella* is a bug that causes nausea, vomiting, diarrhea, and severe stomach cramps that can last for up to two weeks. This workhorse of Microbes Inc. has adapted to survive and proliferate in many foods, but first and foremost in chickens and eggs. Throughout history there has been a direct link between *Salmonella* in poultry and illness in people. Chickens have been supplying a large part of the world's protein for centuries. Traditionally they were raised in small backyard plots and required minimal care, but through overbreeding and mass production the domestic species have become highly susceptible to infections, including the deadly avian influenza virus. Chickens can also carry bugs that lie dormant in their systems but can cause severe illness in people. Primary among these bugs are the many strains of the bacteria *Salmonella*.

With the move to large-scale commercial poultry operations, particularly in Western countries, the threat of *Salmonella* has become an economic as well as a human health issue. *Salmonella* spreads rapidly through high-density chicken barns, and in some places most, if not all, the chickens carry the bacteria from the time they are a few days old. Initially farmers responded to the bacterial threat by providing poultry with antibiotics in their feed. This measure eliminated some forms of *Salmonella* and helped prevent illness in the flocks, but the managers of Microbes Inc. evolved to develop new strains of *Salmonella* that were resistant to antibiotics. The bugs have also adapted to the poultry's systems, so while these strains do not cause illness in chickens, they do affect humans, with sometimes terrible results. And now when people get sick from eating undercooked chicken, it is much more difficult to treat. Every year in North America thousands of infections are directly related to poultry when stringent cooking and cleaning requirements are not met.

*Salmonella* can also colonize eggs, causing severe human illness if they are eaten raw or undercooked. In the 1960s several large outbreaks of a specific kind of salmonella called

*Salmonella enteriditis*, were traced back to eggshells that had been contaminated with bird feces when the eggs were laid. Governments worked with the poultry industry to ensure that eggs were washed and sanitized before they could be commercially sold. But in 1978 and into the early 1980s *S. enteriditis* took off again. This time the infections and outbreaks were associated with clean, unbroken eggs. Scientists finally determined that the eggs were being contaminated by the hens during the incubation process. The crafty *S. enteriditis* bug had found a new way to infect the yolks, which meant that any egg that wasn't cooked thoroughly was a potential health risk. Popular menu items such as hollandaise sauce and Caesar salad dressing were now potentially deadly. In 2009 in the United States alone more than seventy billion eggs are consumed each year, which has resulted in tens of thousands of people becoming ill with this strain of *Salmonella*.

In 1953 a large salmonella outbreak infected more than nine thousand people in Sweden, and caused several fatalities. In response the government, the poultry industry, and consumer groups established a food safety initiative called From Feed to Food, which was designed to prevent *Salmonella* contamination in all parts of the production chain. Poultry operations in Sweden have strict restrictions on where farmers can purchase breeder chickens, on where and how they house the poultry, and on the food and water they provide the birds. Flocks are tested regularly for disease, as are the meat and eggs that go to market — all in an effort to protect consumers from the many strains of *Salmonella*. And it has worked.

By the 1980s Sweden had virtually eliminated *Salmonella* from poultry, and rates of disease in humans followed suit. While the rest of the world was seeing a rise of *S. enteriditis*, Sweden's rate of disease hovered around three in a hundred thousand people, a fraction of the illness reported in most other countries. These measures helped improve food safety, but they are not a panacea. Other bacteria can contaminate poultry, and many other food sources are still vulnerable to *Salmonella* contamination. But rates of infection in Swedes are still much lower than in countries that haven't managed their poultry industry to the same degree. Indeed, Sweden experienced its first large outbreak of salmonella in 2007, shortly after the country joined the European Union, with its less restrictive regulations for poultry production. Seven flocks were infected, and more than a hundred thousand chickens were culled. This frightening incident was summed up in a news release from the Ministry of Agriculture that read, "Poultry producers and processors cannot be too vigilant in preventing pathogens like *Salmonella* from infecting poultry flocks and later ending up on dinner plates."

So why aren't all countries adopting the feed-to-food approach? Mostly because the program is costly to set up and run, and there is still a prevailing attitude — in the United States in particular — that can be summed up in the age-old saying "Buyer beware." We know that properly handling and cooking raw meat can prevent infections, but reducing the upfront risk would certainly benefit society as a whole. The reality is that we aren't all perfect all the time, so anything we can do to stack the odds in our favour is probably a good thing. We should actively encourage government regulators to improve the safety of the food we consume, but we also need to make sure we cook poultry and eggs properly and wash our hands after handling them.

*Salmonella* is a versatile bug, and eliminating it from one food source will not stop it from contaminating others. Chocolate is a particularly intriguing example of the bacteria's remarkable ability to adapt and survive. *Salmonella* has been known to contaminate chocolate since the 1960s, but it wasn't until the 1970s that the first large outbreaks were recorded. In 1970 a large outbreak that affected 110 people in Sweden was traced back to contaminated cocoa powder used in the chocolate products. From December 1973 to February 1974 more than two hundred people, mostly children, in twenty-three American states and seven Canadian provinces contracted a rare strain of *Salmonella* called *S. eastbourne*. Disease detectives in both countries worked tirelessly to trace the origin of the outbreak, which turned out to be chocolate balls produced by a plant in Canada for the Christmas season. Lab tests showed that the cocoa beans used in the production of the chocolate balls were contaminated with this rare form of *Salmonella*.

Chocolate is susceptible to *Salmonella* contamination because its mixture of sugar and fat not only provides the bug with a nice environment in which it can grow but also offers some protection from the acid in the human stomach. This means that only a few bugs can cause illness in many people, and because chocolate is a highly popular and therefore widely distributed treat, contamination can spread over large geographic areas. Despite this knowledge, the bug has proven difficult to keep out of chocolate plants. In 1982, 272 people became ill in England and Wales from contaminated Italian chocolate; hundreds were infected in Canada in 1986 after eating chocolate coins from Belgium; and between October 2001 and March 2002, 439 people in Denmark, Austria, Belgium, the Netherlands, Sweden, Finland, and as far away as Canada fell ill from consuming contaminated chocolate products from a German manufacturer.

Undoubtedly some large outbreaks have been averted by vigilant and regular testing at plants. For example, after three people became ill in the United Kingdom in June 2006, Cadbury recalled more than one million chocolate bars. In November 2006 the Hershey's plant in Ontario was closed down for complete cleaning and disinfection after *Salmonella* was detected in samples; 45,000 kilograms of chocolate were recalled.

Chocolate is not the only processed food that *Salmonella* has effectively targeted. In September 2008 disease trackers in the United States started seeing a spike in illnesses across the country that was caused by a strain of *Salmonella* called *S. typhimurium*. They quickly traced the origins of the disease to a peanut processing plant in Georgia that produced peanut butter and peanut paste used in over four hundred different food products, from cookies to crackers to energy bars and even pet food, that were distributed all across North America. Despite the fact that all of these products were recalled, by early 2009 more than six hundred people had become ill in forty-four states and across Canada. More than half of those who were infected were children, and at least eight people died. And these cases are just the ones we know about. Some estimates suggest that for every person who is diagnosed with salmonella infection, there are as many as thirty-eight others who go undetected or unreported. Tragically, the peanut products outbreak could have been prevented. The company had detected traces of *Salmonella* during routine testing but had chosen not to stop production, find the source of the contamination, and disinfect all the equipment. The company is now under criminal investigation.

These are only a few examples of the havoc caused by *Salmonella*, a highly adaptable bug that can survive in a variety of food products from fresh fruits, nuts, and vegetables to meat, fish, poultry, and processed foods. No wonder this bacteria is the leading cause of food- and water-borne infection. But it is not alone.

## Campylobacter

*Campylobacter*, or "campy," as it is called colloquially, is a bacteria that thrives in many of the same foods as *Salmonella*, especially poultry, eggs, and raw milk. Campy also causes a similar illness to *Salmonella*, with symptoms such as stomach cramps, fever, and diarrhea that can last for a few days to a week. For many years the bacteria surpassed *Salmonella* as the number-one cause of food-borne illness. But outbreaks related to campy infection have not been tracked as closely as some of the other food-borne bacteria. In addition, *Campylobacter* often works in tandem with other bacteria. A classic example was the massive outbreak of illness in Walkerton, Ontario, in 2000. More than 2,300 people in this small community experienced severe gastroenteritis (diarrhea, vomiting, and abdominal cramps) between May and June of that year. Sixty-five people were admitted to hospital, twenty-seven developed the potentially deadly HUS, and seven people died.

An investigation led by a team of disease detectives traced the outbreak back to the municipal water system, which was contaminated with E. coli 0151:H7 and *Campylobacter*. The investigators drew detailed maps, tracking who, where, and when people were becoming ill and modelling the areas around the six wells that supplied the town's drinking water. Their work was based on the investigations that John Snow had conducted in London, England, in the 1850s.

What the disease detectives uncovered was a series of events that had conspired to contaminate the water. First, the town's wells were drilled into groundwater in fields surrounding the town, most of which were being used for cattle. In the days before the outbreak there had been unusually heavy rains. Manure from the cattle had leached into the area around two of the wells. Later the investigators discovered the same *Campylobacter* and E. coli species found in the cattle had leached into the town's drinking water. The water was being monitored by two brothers who worked for the town utilities. Neither of them had been properly trained, and they failed to alert authorities when tests came back positive for contamination. In addition, the chlorination system that helped protect the water from such disease had been on the fritz for several days.

This sad series of events led to the second-largest waterborne outbreak in history and affected the lives and health of thousands. But the tragedy did renew the government's interest in improving and enhancing regulations around drinking-water systems — regulations that had given way to complacency since major health gains had been established a century before, when water safety systems were first developed.

*Campylobacter* not only causes severe diarrhea, fever, and cramps but is also one of the few bacteria that can have lasting effects even after the gastroenteritis clears. In some cases the bug can cause a paralyzing illness called Guillain-Barré syndrome. Others suffer from long-term effects on the joints, which can develop into arthritis. *Campylobacter* lives in the intestines of many animals, including household pets and even birds, and is a common cause of sporadic illness when food, water, or juices have been contaminated by a small amount of animal feces. Outbreaks of the disease have been traced back

122 · DR. BONNIE HENRY

to unpasteurized milk and juice, undercooked eggs and chicken, and raw milk cheeses. The key to prevention is to avoid drinking unpasteurized milk or juice and untreated groundwater, as well as cooking eggs and poultry thoroughly. And always wash your hands after handling raw food.

## Shigella

Third in line after *Salmonella* and *Campylobacter* in causing food- and water-borne illness is a bacterium called *Shigella*. This bug was discovered more than a hundred years ago by Japanese scientist Kiyoshi Shiga. In 1896 Shiga discovered this new bug, which was eventually named after him, while he was tracking the origins of a large dysentery outbreak in Japan. We now know there are several types of shigella, including *S. sonnei* and *S. flexneri*, which are primarily responsible for causing a milder form of disease in developed countries, and *S. dysenteriae*, which still causes massive epidemics in the developing world. *Shigella* affects only humans and primates; most other animals are immune to its nasty effects.

People contract *Shigella* when they consume food or drink that has been contaminated with animal feces — and just a drop will do. It takes as little as ten of these microscopic creatures to cause illness. *Shigella* is commonly passed from soiled hands to mouths (toddlers, with their innate oral curiosity, are at particular risk of contracting the bug this way) and by contaminated foods prepared with unwashed hands. Even fresh fruits and vegetables grown in fields and fertilized with natural products can carry traces of sewage or manure containing this bug.

In 1985 a massive outbreak of *Shigella* infection spread to more than five thousand people in Texas. Disease detectives traced the offending bug back to chopped bagged lettuce that was prepared for a chain of Mexican restaurants across the state. One of the plant workers had become ill with *Shigella*, and poor hygiene practices led to the contamination of thousands of pounds of salad. The lettuce was labelled "ready-to-use," but had the receiving restaurants washed the greens before using them, the unfortunate incident could have been avoided.

Similar outbreaks in Norway, Sweden, and the United Kingdom in the late 1990s affected hundreds who became ill after eating iceberg lettuce from Spain. And two decades after the Texas outbreak, people across North America contracted the disease after eating prepackaged spinach laced with *Shigella*. In both cases the cleaning process at the packaging plant had not removed all of the offending bugs, despite the fact that the products were labelled "prewashed" and "ready-to-use."

Leafy vegetables are not the only food associated with this bacteria. *Shigella* has also been associated with chopped turkey, rice balls, beans, pudding, fresh strawberries, raw oysters, deli meats, and unpasteurized milk. In 2002 almost a thousand people became ill in central and eastern Canada after eating commercially prepared Greek-style pasta salad. The salad was prepared in bulk in Ontario and distributed to grocery stores, restaurants, and cafeterias in schools and hospitals across half the country. Hundreds of people became ill, including seven hundred in Ontario alone. This outbreak was also traced back to an infected person who prepared the bulk salad and whose hygiene habits were not up to scratch. As with many food-borne bacteria, the key to prevention is by washing produce, cooking meat thoroughly, and adhering to good hand-hygiene practices.

## E. coli and the Rise of Hamburger Disease

No discussion of food-related diseases would be complete without including a bug that went from benign to deadly in just a few decades. It starts with the story of cattle and the evolution of the beef industry, and it ends on the dinner plate.

*Escherichia coli* O157:H7, or E. coli, is one of the most famous and deadly bugs to be associated with beef. E. coli has been living symbiotically in the human intestine for centuries, but in the late 1980s a new strain of the bacteria emerged that was eventually given the scientific name E. coli O157:H7. The bug made its dramatic entry into the world's consciousness in 1993, when a large outbreak was traced back to hamburgers served at Jack in the Box fast food restaurants in the American Pacific Northwest. Almost seven hundred people were hospitalized with bloody diarrhea, fevers, and severe abdominal cramps, and a hundred people, mostly children, developed HUS. Four children died.

While this incident may have marked the bacterium's grand public debut, in reality E. coli O157:H7 had been quietly lurking in our environment for several decades. A Swiss pediatrician first described hemolytic uremic syndrome in 1955; it was occurring in his young patients. At the time the disease wasn't linked to any bacterium, but we now know that HUS is a hallmark of damage caused by the toxin-producing E. coli O157:H7. E. coli in its more benign form was first described by the German pediatrician Theodore Escherich in 1885. For the past century scientists considered E. coli one of the good bugs, part of the human body's normal flora that help with digestion and fight off disease-causing bugs. When this new O157:H7 strain was found in 1975 in the stool of a woman from California suffering from a severe case of bloody diarrhea, most scientists thought this form of the bacteria was just a curious anomaly. The samples were relegated to the storage shelves of the U.S. CDC in Atlanta, Georgia.

Seven years later an outbreak of a particularly nasty gastrointestinal illness was traced back to hamburgers served at McDonald's restaurants in Oregon and Michigan. Disease investigators from the CDC dug into the vaults and soon realized it was the same strain that had made the woman in California ill. This outbreak did not attract much attention, which allowed the nasty bug to expand its reach. In 1985 an outbreak in a nursing home in London, Ontario, killed seventeen residents. An outbreak among Inuit in Canada's Northwest Territories infected more than five hundred people over several months in 1991; twenty-two people developed HUS and two died. Despite these alarming outbreaks, most public health officials and laboratory scientists still considered E. coli O157:H7 a rare variation of a generally good bug. But the evidence was mounting, and outbreaks of disease in 1991 from unpasteurized apple cider that had been contaminated by cattle manure started to raise alarms. But it took the sheer magnitude of the Jack in the Box outbreak to put this bug into the public lexicon for good. The multi-state epidemic even spawned the moniker "hamburger disease." So how did this all happen?

It is likely that the E. coli bug evolved over the past fifty thousand years by picking up viruses that allowed the bacterium to escape the immune systems of animals and humans. Over time the O157:H7 strain became proficient at picking up new pieces of genetic material and gained a selective advantage over other members of the E. coli family. At some point the E. coli O157:H7 bug picked up a piece of virus DNA that allowed it to produce a toxin that acts like a vicious hooligan in the human gut, attacking the stomach lining and the red cells and platelets in the blood. The toxin causes large ulcers, bleeding, and severe cramping. In some people, especially children and the elderly, the toxin can attack the small blood vessels in the kidneys, leading to clots that cut off the blood supply to these vital organs. HUS develops when the kidneys can no longer function to clean the blood of toxins, leading to a cascade of damage to the other organs that can be deadly.

When scientists first investigated the toxin after E. coli O157:H7's world debut, they found that it looked and acted like the toxin found in Shigella, another bug that causes severe bloody diarrheal illness in people, so it was classified as a Shiga toxin. But just having the toxin wasn't enough to make this bug a real contender; there were a few other variables that led to the spread of the bacteria's destructive powers. E. coli O157:H7 and other toxin-producing E. coli strains proved to be the product of affluent industrialized countries — countries that can afford to feed antibiotics to cattle and other livestock to enhance their growth.

In the 1950s farmers began feeding their cattle small doses of antibiotics to spur growth in the animals. At the time they were unaware of the negative impact this practice would have on the normal flora that had lived in the animals' guts for centuries. The antibiotics killed the good bugs and allowed some strains, such as O157:H7, to develop resistance to the drugs and thrive. Somewhere along the way, E. coli O157:H7 also acquired the ability to withstand the acid environment of the human stomach. And as with Shigella, ingesting only a few hundred of the organisms can make someone ill. But even these characteristics — producing a virulent toxin, the ability to grow in antibiotic-fed cattle, the ability to resist the stomach's acid environment — were not enough; it took the workings of humans to build the perfect storm that led to the hamburger disease tragedy.

The industrialization of the beef industry gave E. coli O157:H7 its stairway to the world stage. Cattle in most industrialized countries are now raised in hundreds of highly efficient but crowded feedlots with centralized food, water, and waste management systems. This practice exposes thousands of animals to bugs such as E. coli O157:H7, and once they are exposed, these bugs take over the guts of upwards of 60 percent of the animals. When the cattle reach their optimal size and weight, they are transported by the thousands to centralized slaughterhouses that often service several dozen feedlots. From there the carcasses are transferred to plants that separate the meat from the bone, and then large bins of raw beef are sent to processing plants. To make hamburger, bins of meat from many plants are fed into gigantic grinders; it is then formed mechanically into patties, which are frozen before being sent out to the world. This large-scale industrial process is nirvana for bugs such as E. coli O157:H7. Even a small amount of bacteria can contaminate hundreds of thousands of pounds of hamburger meat. In the case of the Jack in the Box outbreak in 1993, scientists estimate that the hamburger patties contained meat from 443 different cattle that came from farms in six states and from five slaughterhouses.

The Jack in the Box scandal occurred during the company's promotion of its new Monster Burger, which was advertised as a larger, thicker patty. The outbreak could have been avoided had the meat been thoroughly cooked, and it gave a whole new meaning to the company's promotional slogan, "Tastes so good it's scary." Hamburger has a particularly high risk of containing bacteria such as E. coli O157:H7 because the bugs tend to be well mixed throughout the meat. These bacteria, however, can be killed by high temperatures — at least 71°C (160°F). For hamburger this translates into cooking the meat until it's well done. Other cuts of beef are also at risk of being contaminated with bacteria, but in the case of roasts, steaks, or filets the bugs generally remain on the surface of the meat, so often a brief searing will reach the requisite temperature to kill the bugs, which is why a rare steak does not pose the same risk of causing illness as undercooked hamburger. Yet even with this knowledge, some restaurants still advertise with pride burgers that are pink in the middle!

As for E. coli O157:H7, since its Jack in the Box days this nasty bug continues to be a cause of outbreaks affecting thousands and has been linked to a variety of food sources. These include beef jerky, dry salami, and roast beef that was found to be contaminated after cooking, as well as bean sprouts, lettuce, broccoli, fallen apples, unpasteurized juice, and unpasteurized milk, proving that the sometimes severe disease caused by this emerging strain has spread well beyond hamburger meat.

## Milk Madness

In recent years unpasteurized milk has become trendy in some affluent areas of Canada and the United States. Many have clearly forgotten or are wilfully blind to the lessons of the past that led to the development and widespread use of pasteurization in the first place. As its name suggests, the process of pasteurization was invented by the French chemist and bacteriologist Louis Pasteur in 1862. At the time Pasteur was looking for a way to protect wine from spoilage, but the process was soon recognized as an important and effective way to kill the bacteria, parasites, and spores in raw milk. Originally the milk was heated to just below the boiling point to kill the offending microbes without curdling it. The most common method used today is called high-temperature–short-time pasteurization. The milk is rapidly heated to 71.7°C (161°F) for just fifteen to twenty seconds. This process does not sterilize the milk but is designed to kill a sufficient number of organisms for safe consumption, generally 99.999 percent, or a five-log reduction.

More important, this process is effective at killing heat-resistant bugs such as *Mycobacterium tuberculosis*, which causes TB, and *Coxiella burnetii*, which causes an illness known as Q fever, a disease characterized by fever, coughing, and gastrointestinal illness that can even lead to death. With the advent of pasteurization, illnesses such as these have all but disappeared, and other common bugs such as *Salmonella*, *Shigella*, and E. coli (even E. coli O157:H7), which historically caused illness in many and even death in some, are no longer a risk of drinking milk. So how can we explain the movement in some areas back towards drinking raw milk?

There is no scientific evidence that raw milk contains more vitamins, is more nutritious, or even tastes better than unpasteurized milk; indeed, the only thing raw milk has more of is bugs. Blind taste tests have shown that people cannot tell the difference between raw and pasteurized milk. The raw milk trend can only be explained as a nostalgic return to what is thought to be a simpler time, when milk was obtained from the local farmer and there were no E. coli O157 strains lurking in the environment. The unfortunate thing is that the lessons the leaders of Microbes Inc. taught us in the past seem to have been forgotten among so many today.

## Listeria and Luncheon Meats

We cannot leave the Bacteria Division without considering perhaps the most notorious member of Microbes Inc. to be associated with processed foods: *Listeria monocytogenes*. *Listeria* was first described by the British veterinarian and microbiologist E. D. G. Murray in 1926, after he determined the bacteria was the cause of fatal illness in eight rabbits. Murray named the bug *Bacterium monocytogenes*, but in 1940 scientist Harvey Pirie changed the name to *Listeria monocytogenes* in honour of Joseph Lister, the pioneer of disinfection.

Several reports were published in the 1920s detailing a clinical disease caused by *Listeria* in animals and humans. But it wasn't until 1952 that *Listeria* was recognized as a serious cause of meningitis, an infection of the lining of the brain, and sepsis, an infection in the blood, in newborns in East Germany. It was later found to also cause disease in adults whose immune systems were compromised by conditions such as HIV infection, chronic illness, or treatment for cancers. We now know that the illness listeriosis can lead to spontaneous abortion or stillbirth in pregnant women and is a major cause of meningitis in newborn babies. In adults the disease most often causes intestinal infections that lead to nausea, diarrhea, abdominal cramping, and headaches; in rare adult cases the infection can cause sepsis or meningitis. Listeriosis is an opportunistic disease that takes advantage of the vulnerable, and as a result it has the highest mortality rates of any food-borne illness.

*Listeria* was virtually unknown before the production of ready-to-eat foods. The first recorded outbreak of the disease was in Halifax, Nova Scotia, in 1981. Forty-one people, mostly pregnant women and young children, became ill, and eighteen died from the disease. The bacteria were traced back to mass-produced coleslaw containing cabbage that had been contaminated by sheep manure. Since then *Listeria* has been found in many ready-to-eat foods, from hot dogs and deli meats to soft cheeses, smoked fish, and pâté.

In the late summer of 2008 *Listeria* was the cause of an outbreak in Ontario that was traced back to a giant Maple Leaf Foods plant in Toronto. Its popular ready-to-eat deli meats were shipped to restaurants, grocery stores, and institutions such as hospitals across the country. More than two hundred products were recalled, and the outbreak resulted in twenty-three deaths in seven provinces. Later the investigation of this tragedy revealed the difficulties in keeping *Listeria* out of even the cleanest processing plants.

*Listeria* is a hardy bacterium that lives in soil, vegetation, water, sewage, and the feces of both animals and humans. Over the years the bug has evolved to be able to thrive in temperatures as low as 0°C (32°F). This means that the bacteria can grow in most refrigerators, which are set at around 4°C (39°F), a temperature that usually stops the growth of or kills most bacteria. So if you put a package of sliced ham, for example, in your refrigerator for a week, even a small amount of *Listeria* can grow in these conditions and make you sick. But, like other food-borne bugs, *Listeria* is sensitive to heat, so cooking or steaming foods will rapidly kill the bacteria. The peril of ready-to-eat products, however, is that for the most part they don't require cooking.

Most people are frequently exposed to low levels of *Listeria* but don't get sick because their immune systems can handle the bug. Those with weakened immune systems, however, need to be careful about avoiding high-risk foods or ensuring they are cooked. In addition, washing your hands after handling fresh produce and raw meat and cleaning your kitchen counters and cutting boards are important measures to combat *Listeria* — and all the other bugs that thrive in ready-to-eat foods.

## Food, Bugs, and Climate Change: *Vibrio parahaemolyticus*

The final bacterium we will look at is one that grows in the ocean. A gradual increase in the temperature of the world's oceans has had some interesting effects on the food we eat. On average, temperatures in the northern oceans have warmed by one to three degrees in the past hundred years. This increase might not seem dramatic but it has had an impact on the bugs that live in the oceans and on the fish and shellfish we eat.

One compelling example of the impact of global warming and increasing ocean temperatures is the emergence of the bacterium *Vibrio parahaemolyticus* in the northern waters off the coast of British Columbia and Washington State. These cold waters are the perfect environment for the cultivation of oysters. But in the past few years there have been several reports of disease in people who have consumed raw oysters, and local public health officials traced these outbreaks back to the coastal oyster beds, areas that previously were thought not to be warm enough for the bacteria to grow.

*Vibrio parahaemolyticus,* a cousin to the bug that causes cholera, lives in salt water only and thrives when water temperatures rise. In many places this means during the summer months — May, June, July, and August — which may have given rise to the sage advice never to eat raw oysters in months without an R in them. *Vibrio* is a bacterium that causes an intestinal infection, the symptoms of which include explosive watery diarrhea and abdominal cramps that usually start within twelve to twenty-four hours of eating the contaminated food. In most people the illness lasts only two to three days, but in some the infection can be more severe, causing high fever, bloody diarrhea, and dehydration that can last for as long as a week. Rarely, however, do people die from this infection.

About 4,500 cases of illness from *Vibrio parahaemolyticus* are reported in the United States every year, but this is likely the tip of the iceberg, since most infections are short-lived and often people don't bother to visit their doctor or report their symptoms. When cases are reported, the illness is most often traced back to consumption of raw or undercooked fish and shellfish, especially oysters. In 2007 fifteen cases of *Vibrio* were reported in British Columbia, and all of them were traced back to raw oysters — most were from oysters served at some of the fanciest restaurants in the area!

Shellfish are an excellent source of protein and are high in essential minerals and low in calories, fat, and cholesterol. Oysters, clams, scallops, and mussels are all commonly found and cultivated in salt water, and all are sensitive to their marine environment. Luckily, as with many of the infections we have discussed, cooking shellfish thoroughly kills *Vibrio parahaemolyticus*. The other way to protect your health is to make sure you refrigerate or freeze shellfish until you are ready to eat it, so the bugs don't have a chance to grow. And, of course, always wash your hands after handling raw seafood.

## VIRUSES

While bacteria may rule the world of food-borne illnesses, theirs is not the only division of Microbes Inc. that has adapted to our food and water supply. There are also a few major players from the Virus Division of this global corporation. For the most part they cause illnesses that are more rapid in onset and shorter-lived.

### Norovirus

The most common food-borne virus is a new player on the scene, one that causes a short but nasty illness characterized by explosive vomiting, stomach cramps, and watery diarrhea, and it goes by the name of Norovirus. The Norovirus was originally called Norwalk virus after the town in Ohio where it made its debut in 1968, causing illness in a school full of elementary students. The virus itself was discovered in 1972, and since then it has been found around the world. It has garnered the nickname "winter vomiting disease," for the season it tends to strike in most often, and has been associated with an innumerable variety of foods, from pizza to salad greens to shellfish. The virus also gained international notoriety for attacking vacationers on cruise ships — not a pleasant way to spend a vacation!

Noroviruses are small and very contagious; only a few hundred bugs can cause illness. Both the stool and vomit of infected people contain millions of the tiny organisms, which can remain active in human waste for several days. Most people get sick by eating food or drinking fluids that have been tainted with the virus. Transmission commonly occurs when contaminated people neglect to wash their hands after using the toilet or caring for someone who is ill and then prepare food. The disease usually comes on suddenly, with severe vomiting that often leads to heavy contamination of the environment. Many have contracted the disease just by touching contaminated surfaces that haven't been thoroughly cleaned. Despite the dramatic nature of the illness, most people recover fully within twenty-four to forty-eight hours.

Prevention of this sneaky virus goes back to the basics of hygiene. Always wash your hands carefully after using the toilet and before preparing or eating food. And if someone in your household does become ill, clean up all surfaces thoroughly with a solution that consists of one part household bleach to nine parts water. People who prepare food at restaurants or for large groups should not work when they are ill and should stay home for at least two or three days after the symptoms stop. Most health departments require restaurants to follow these safety regulations, but sometimes people fall through the cracks, as we have seen again and again, and the results can be devastating.

## Hepatitis A

The other common food- and water-borne virus is one that affects the liver: hepatitis A. Unlike its cousins hepatitis B, C, and D, which are mostly passed on through blood, this virus spreads through contaminated food and water. With our improved sanitation systems and safe drinking water, this bug is rarely a threat in most Western countries. It is, however, an important cause of travel-related illness in countries where meeting sanitation standards is still a challenge.

Most hepatitis A outbreaks in North America in the past decade have been linked to imported produce that was tainted with sewage in the fields. One particularly large outbreak affected schoolchildren in California, who contracted the disease from fresh strawberries that were part of their school lunch program. The strawberries hadn't been washed sufficiently before the students ate them. In 2003 the then-largest hepatitis A outbreak recorded in the United States involved more than six hundred people who ate at a restaurant in Pittsburgh, Pennsylvania; three people died. Disease detectives traced the source of the outbreak back to raw green onions that were served at the restaurant; the onions had been imported from Mexico. This tragic outbreak came on the heels of smaller outbreaks in Tennessee, North Carolina, and Georgia earlier that year, which caused illness in 422 people and were also linked to imported green onions from Mexico.

Along with observing good hygiene practices and washing or cooking fresh produce thoroughly, another effective way to prevent hepatitis A is through vaccination. Following the tragic outbreak in Pittsburgh, public health officials started a universal childhood vaccination program across the United States. Other Western countries are now looking closely at adopting the program in order to prevent widespread illness among children, who tend to carry the virus longer than adults do and are therefore more likely to pass infection on to others.

## PARASITES

From *Salmonella* in chickens and eggs to E. coli in beef and dairy cattle and Noroviruses on cruise ships, we have now seen how bacteria and viruses have successfully invaded our food and water systems. Let's see how the Parasite Division of Microbes Inc. has evolved to invade our food and water supply.

## Taming Trichinella

A good place to start is with the parasite *Trichinella*. Originally *Trichinella spiralis* was a very common parasite in pigs. The painful and sometimes fatal disease trichinellosis, is directly linked to eating undercooked contaminated pork. Although the idea is controversial, trichinellosis has been cited by some scholars (along with the pork tapeworm) as the reason behind the prohibition of pork and pork products in Islam and Judaism. Disease associated with pork consumption has been recorded for centuries, well before microbes were identified as the cause. But today this parasite has been virtually eliminated in the Western world through improved animal husbandry practices.

The bug was first recognized in 1835, but it took another decade or so for the American scientist Joseph Leidy to associate the disease caused by this parasite with the consumption of undercooked pork. It took several more decades before this association was widely accepted by the scientific community, in part because *Trichinella* can cause such a wide variety of symptoms, especially in the early stages of disease. Contaminated meat is characterized by cysts that form in the pigs' flesh. Once someone ingests the undercooked meat, the acid in the stomach dissolves the hard outer layer of the cyst, releasing the adult parasite worms. These worms travel to the small intestine, where they mature and eventually release larvae. The larvae then journey through the circulatory system in search of muscle where they can safely hide away for years.

In the early stages of illness people experience nausea, dyspepsia (stomach upset), and diarrhea — the same symptoms caused by a myriad of other bugs. About one to two weeks later the larvae move into the muscles; the symptoms can include headaches, fever, chills, coughing, and eye swelling, along with muscle pain, itching, and skin rash. It takes an astute clinician to consider trichinellosis as the cause — our French hunters were lucky that their consumption of bear meat likely tipped off their doctors.

Just a few decades ago this elusive bug caused hundreds of cases of disease in developed countries, including the United States and Canada. Pigs are not picky eaters and will consume anything from their preferred acorns and nuts to animal and human waste, and everything in between. In the past thirty years most developed countries passed laws that prohibited feeding raw garbage to hogs, in an effort to combat trichinellosis. This practice, along with consumer awareness of the need to cook pork properly, has led to a dramatic decrease in trichinellosis in many parts of the world. In the United States, on average twelve cases are reported every year, some of which are related to the consumption of contaminated meat outside of the country.

But *Trichinella* is still a major problem in many areas of the world, especially in low- and middle-income countries where public food and safety laws have not been enacted. These regions include many Southeast Asian countries, Eastern Europe, and Mexico — countries where over 50 percent of hogs are infected with *Trichinella*. People who travel to these parts of the world need to practise caution to ensure that any pork products they consume are well cooked and properly handled.

In the northern regions of Canada *Trichinella* is present in up to 10 percent of polar bears and walruses, and both of these animals are traditional food sources for the Inuit population. While trichinellosis is now rare in most of Canada, rates of illness in these northern communities are as high as eleven in a hundred thousand people. In 1999 an outbreak of trichinellosis affected thirty-four of the sixty-two Inuit who consumed the delicacy of raw walrus in a single community on Baffin Island. This outbreak led to a study that showed that almost 20 percent of the community of five hundred had antibodies to *Trichinella* in their blood. The presence of these antibodies indicated that the inhabitants had been exposed to the bug at some point in their lives. Preventing trichinellosis in northern communities continues to be an ongoing dilemma: the small but real risk of disease must be weighed against the value of traditional food sources and preparation methods. This is an important example of the sometimes intense cultural and political debate that can erupt around food, pitting safety against tradition.

## Cyclospora

How many people living in Western countries today know exactly where their fresh organic basil purchased at the local grocery store really came from? What about the strawberries at the local market labelled "Product of California"? The truth is, the movement of food across continents and oceans today is mind-boggling. The repackaging, mixing, and mass distribution of food has become so complex that tracing the path of a particular product when something goes wrong has proven exceedingly difficult. And go wrong it does, and sadly on a regular basis. The move towards organic produce — and the higher prices such products can fetch — has led to the development of organic farms in Mexico and South America that ship produce into the United States, Canada, and, less commonly, countries in Europe. Regulations in Canada, as in many countries, allow a product to be labelled "Product of Canada" as long as a portion of it comes from Canadian farms and is packaged in a Canadian facility. Large facilities collect produce from local organic farms, then package and distribute these products to grocery stores in the surrounding area. But when local production is low, the produce is supplemented with organic products from other provinces or countries. But good farming, packaging, and hygiene practices are not always monitored at these facilities. This is what led to an outbreak of the unusual parasite *Cyclospora* in British Columbia.

In the summer of 2007 the growing season for organic basil on farms in British Columbia was delayed by inclement weather in the spring. Basil imported from Mexico made up the shortfall. Within weeks people in British Columbia were reporting symptoms caused by a bug not usually found in Canada, *Cyclospora cayetanensis*. This outbreak got the attention of disease detectives in the province, and a detailed investigation quickly ensued. It can take several days for symptoms from parasites such as *Cyclospora* to surface, and a few more days before people feel unwell enough to see a doctor. If stool cultures are sent for testing, it can take a few more days before the symptoms are diagnosed and the patient receives treatment. By that time health officials are several weeks behind in their investigation, and unfortunately many patients find it difficult to recall in detail what they consumed or where they ate in the days before becoming ill.

During this outbreak public health investigators were granted permission from patients to access product information tracked by their grocery store loyalty cards. This allowed officials to determine exactly what groceries had been purchased when and to see if there were common patterns of purchase and consumption among those who had become ill. This detective work led to the identification of a specific type of organic basil that came from one production facility. Then the fun part began — trying to figure out where the basil was grown and how it had become contaminated.

Tracing the basil's winding trail proved time-consuming and involved local, provincial, and even federal agencies, such is the complexity of our food distribution system. But the trail eventually led to a farm in Mexico that lacked the proper sanitation facilities for its workers. One or more of the farm workers had likely become ill, and because there were no washrooms on site they either passed the bug on to the basil during harvesting or when they relieved themselves in the fields. The plight of poor and migrant farm workers in places such as Mexico, Guatemala, Ecuador, and other low-income countries, as well as the impact of export cash crops such as organic basil, bananas, raspberries, and other fresh produce on their communities, is just beginning to make its way into the consciousness of North Americans. Outbreaks like this one have highlighted the high risk of spreading infection through the global food market.

## TOXINS

The final division of Microbes Inc. that continues to affect our food is a specialized group of bacteria that produce toxins classically associated with certain foods. Most of these toxins cause short-term illness, like that produced by *Bacillus cereus*, which is often found in steamed rice that has been sitting at room temperature for some time. But one has proven to be more severe, and even deadly.

## Botulism

*Trichinella* is not the only bug associated with traditional food preparation in northern communities around the world. In the past three decades botulism has also become a threat to the health of Inuit and other aboriginal communities in Canada and the United States. Botulism is a poisoning caused by a toxin produced by *Clostridium botulinum*, a bacterium that is commonly found in soil worldwide. *C. botulinum* can live nicely in harsh conditions with very little oxygen. The bacteria form hardy spores to protect themselves from these hostile environments and can live in the soil for long periods of time. When they find themselves in a more welcoming environment, the spores germinate and the microbe reproduction cycle starts again.

There are three main types of botulism: food-borne, which is contracted by ingesting contaminated food; wound botulism, which forms when the bacteria infect the bloodstream through cuts or punctures; and infant botulism, which occurs when young babies ingest the spores and the bacteria germinate in the child's intestine, releasing a poisonous toxin. Wound botulism was a cause of many deaths during early wars but has since been quite rare, though the past twenty-five years have seen increasing numbers of cases of wound botulism associated with injecting black tar heroin. It is the food-borne form, however, that is the cause of much of the illness we are seeing in aboriginal communities today.

Botulism has been around for centuries. The disease was called "sausage poisoning" in the eighteenth and nineteenth centuries because of the number of people who contracted the disease from consuming contaminated sausage. The name *botulism* actually comes from the Latin word for sausage, *botulus*. The disease itself was first described in 1897 by a physician named Emile van Ermengem following an investigation of a large outbreak in Ellezelles, Belgium. He described the classic symptoms of blurred or double vision, slurred speech, drooping eyelids, dry mouth, difficulty swallowing, and muscle weakness, which started anywhere from eighteen to thirty-six hours after ingesting contaminated food. These symptoms progressed to paralysis of the legs and arms, then the trunk and respiratory muscles, and could lead to death in as many as half the cases.

Today ventilator support and intensive medical care, along with antitoxin treatment, have reduced the fatality rate of botulism to 3 to 5 percent. An antitoxin made from horse antibodies is available in small amounts worldwide, but a rigorous testing protocol must be followed to ensure that the recipient won't have a deadly reaction to the antitoxin itself. The antitoxin works to stop the progression of the disease by binding to and then inactivating the toxin. Sadly, it doesn't reverse the damage that has already been done. People who have botulism generally require weeks to months of intensive therapy to recover, and many suffer from long-term fatigue and weakness.

Botulism is thankfully rare in most countries these days, with the United States reporting about twenty-five cases each year and Canada ten to twenty cases annually. It is still a much larger problem in other countries, such as the Democratic Republic of Georgia, where hundreds of cases are still reported every year. Most cases are related to the consumption of home-canned goods, especially low-acid foods such as asparagus, green beans, beets, and corn. After the economic meltdown in 2008 there was an increase in reported cases of botulism from improperly home-canned produce as more people began using this method to save on food costs.

By contrast, in the early 1900s large numbers of botulism cases were reported from consumption of commercially canned foods. In the 1920s strict regulations were introduced for commercial canning operations, and since then cases of botulism linked to these products have been much less common. Still, there have on occasion been large outbreaks related to commercially canned foods, including one in 1971 when a man from New York died after eating Bon Vivant canned vichyssoise (a cold potato soup). A massive recall of Bon Vivant products eventually led to the company's collapse. More recently, in the summer of 2007 an outbreak of botulism caused severe illness in eight people across three U.S. states (Indiana, Ohio, and Texas), all of whom had eaten Castleberry's canned chili sauce. Despite strict regulations, mistakes can happen. It is important always to remember to avoid cans that are dented or bloated, as this may be a sign of contamination.

Recognized outbreaks of botulism have also been related to food consumed at restaurants. One of the largest outbreaks on record infected thirty-six people from across North America in 1988; it was traced back to food containing pre-chopped garlic in oil at a restaurant in Vancouver. In 1994 thirty people became sick after eating at a Greek restaurant in Texas. In that case the bacteria were found in baked potatoes that had been wrapped in aluminum foil and left for several days at room temperature before being used in dips. One of the most geographically widespread outbreaks was in the fall of 2006, when one woman in Florida and three people in Georgia developed botulism after drinking organic carrot juice produced in California. The product was recalled globally, and in follow-up investigations public health officials found two people in Toronto and one person in Montreal who had also been hospitalized with botulism after drinking the same carrot juice. This outbreak reminds us just how widespread the distribution of food has become.

Despite these highly publicized outbreaks, the largest number of cases of botulism in the United States and Canada in the past twenty years has been concentrated in aboriginal and Inuit communities. A review of Inuit and First Nations people in Canada between 1980 and 2009 uncovered fifty-eight reported incidents of consumption of botulism-laced foods, which led to 119 cases of illness and twenty-two deaths. This is in stark contrast to non-Native cases: in the same time period nine incidents were reported, leading to forty-six cases of illness and only a single death. The Inuit and First Nations cases were linked to traditional foods such as raw whale, seal, walrus, char, and caribou meat, and fermented fish, salmon eggs, and muktuk. The higher death rates in these cases are most likely due to a combination of delayed recognition of the illness and the remote location of many Inuit communities, making timely access to medical care difficult to provide.

Reports from Alaska mirror the findings in Canada. Fifty-eight botulism outbreaks were documented in the state between 2004 and 2009, and 103 people, almost all native Alaskans, were affected by the disease. Between 1990 and 2000 ninety-seven cases of botulism were caused by one of the seven toxin types — toxin E — and ninety-one of the cases were in native Alaskans. Toxin E is the type most associated with marine mammals, and the majority of the ill had contracted the infection from consumption of traditionally prepared animals. The toxin can be destroyed by cooking, but many traditional native foods are served raw or go through a process of fermentation in order to preserve the texture and flavour of the meat.

So how can we balance the cultural importance and health benefits of traditional aboriginal and Inuit foods while addressing the slight but real risk of botulism? It turns out that some factors have changed over the past thirty years that could account for the increased risk of botulism in native communities. The traditional preparation of foods such as muktuk (fermented seal or beluga whale) or the preparation of mikiyak (fermented whale meat, blubber, and skin in seal oil), tipmuk (fermented fish), stink eggs (fermented salmon eggs), and stink heads (fermented fish heads) involved burying the meat or fish in pits, which were often layered with willow leaves, for one to two weeks until the meat putrefied. This method allowed for circulation of air and prevented the growth of C. botulinum. Since the 1970s the dramatic increase of botulism outbreaks from these same foods has had a direct correlation to the development of plastic containers and resealable plastic bags. These modern containers create an anaerobic (low-oxygen) environment that kills off most bacteria but provides perfect conditions for C. botulinum to thrive.

An outbreak of botulism in western Alaska in 2002 exposed this phenomenon. In July of that year two hunters from a Yupik community came across a beached beluga whale that they estimated had been there for several weeks. Following their centuries-old traditions they cut the meat away from the whale's fluke to share with members of their village. Untraditionally, however, they stored the meat in sealed plastic bags, which were then kept in the refrigerator before being consumed by the hunters and their families a few days later. Of the fourteen people who consumed the whale meat, eight contracted severe cases of botulism and two required the support of a ventilator.

Luckily, Alaskan public health officials had recognized the increased risk of botulism in the area and had implemented an extensive education and awareness program to diagnose early-stage illness and rapidly provide medical care for the sick. They had also stockpiled antitoxin in the rural medical centres so treatment could begin immediately. All fourteen survived the outbreak, but the incident highlighted the risk of mixing modern conveniences with the preparation of traditional foods. There is an ongoing effort to educate Inuit and Native community leaders about these potential health risks and to encourage a return to traditional methods of food preparation. The example of botulism offers hard evidence that new and modern is not always better when it comes to bugs and food.

❧

IN OUR SEARCH for cheap, tasty, and nutritional sources of sustenance combined with our insatiable desire for fresh seasonal foods all year round, we have created increasingly complex and wide-reaching networks that have allowed bugs to thrive and to spread globally. There are trade-offs involved with all the things we do to meet our modern needs and desires. If we don't use antibiotics on cattle, for example, it takes more time and energy to raise the animals, requires more land, and creates more waste. On the other hand, the use of these drugs has been associated with a dramatic increase in potentially deadly antibiotic-resistant bugs in our environment.

Governments need to look at modern options such as limiting the amount and the types of antibiotics used in animals to bring the balance back towards human health. As Albert Einstein wisely observed, "No problem can be solved from the same level of consciousness that created it. We must learn to think anew." Certainly the divisions of Microbes Inc. are continually thinking anew, evolving to overcome our attempts to keep them out of our food and happily taking advantage of the weaknesses in our global food production and distribution systems. Gone are the days when most people grew their own fruits and vegetables or bought them from the local farmer's market. If a product was contaminated with a bacteria or virus twenty years ago, chances are only a small local outbreak would occur. But today's large farms, coupled with North American and European consumer expectations, mean that we can find produce from all over the world, at any time of year, in our local big-box grocery store. There has always been an inherent risk of contracting illness from fresh fruits and vegetables, but now we have to be concerned about new bugs from many areas of the world.

While the risk is ever-changing, the best ways to protect ourselves remain the same: washing fruits and vegetables carefully before consumption and cleaning our hands both before and after handling foods can greatly reduce the risk of contamination. Other important measures include refrigerating produce after cutting it up to prevent the growth of bacteria, and cooking meat, seafood, and vegetables, which will effectively kill most bugs.

If your immune system is compromised for any reason, there are some foods you should probably avoid unless they are cooked. These include all kinds of sprouts, which can be contaminated in the seed and are virtually impossible to wash clean; ready-to-eat luncheon meats; and unpasteurized milk and cheeses, to name a few. Governments in Western countries have developed programs in cooperation with low-income countries to help improve the sanitation and living conditions of farming communities, as a way of reducing the risk at the source. These programs are part of an evolving "farm to fork" approach to food safety, and while they help, they do not negate the need to wash your hands and your produce at home as well.

From processed cold cuts to the veggies we grow in our own back garden, nothing we eat is 100 percent safe from the world of Microbes Inc. All foods and drinks have the potential to make us sick if we are not careful and do not follow a few simple rules: Eat locally as often as you can. Wash your hands before preparing and eating food. Wash your countertops and cutting boards after preparing foods. A good solution consists of 1 teaspoon of bleach in 3 cups of water: spray the cleaner on the cutting board, let it stand for a few minutes, then wash off with warm water. Wash all fruits and vegetables thoroughly, especially if you eat them raw. Organic does not mean your food is bug free! Organic produce still needs to be washed and cooked thoroughly to prevent infections. Don't eat raw meat or drink raw milk; it is just not worth the risk. Be aware of and abide by safe cooking temperatures (see p. 150). And wash your hands, wash your hands, wash your hands! At the end of the day the number-one way bugs get into our bodies is from our hands to our mouth.

As we have seen, our food production and distribution systems continue to evolve and increase in complexity and scope. The bugs of Microbes Inc. continue to adapt to these changes and find ways to exploit any lapses or gaps in our food safety networks. In the end, prevention is key and following these few simple measures is still our best protection.

### SAFE COOKING TEMPERATURES

You can't tell by looking—use a food thermometer to be sure!

| FOOD | TEMPERATURE |
|---|---|
| beef/veal steaks and roasts | |
| medium-rare | 63°C (145°F) |
| medium | 71°C (160°F) |
| well done | 77°C (170°F) |
| ground beef/pork/veal | 71°C (160°F) |
| food made with ground beef/ | |
| pork/veal (e.g., sausages, meatballs) | |
| pork chops, ribs, roasts | 74°C (165°F) |
| ground chicken/turkey | |
| food made with ground chicken/ | |
| turkey (e.g. sausages, meatballs) | |
| chicken/turkey breasts, legs, thighs, and wings | |
| stuffing, casseroles, hot dogs, leftovers, egg dishes | |
| chicken/turkey (whole, unstuffed) | 85°C (185°F) |

# FIVE

# BUGS IN THE
# NEIGHBOURHOOD

I N SEPTEMBER 2000 a doctor in Watsonville, California, saw
his fourth patient in as many weeks with strange boils on
her legs. Something unusual was going on. All four women
had painful red, oozing lumps on their lower legs, and with
this last case he discovered that they had all had a pedicure
in the days before the sores appeared. He called his local
public health officer to look into the matter further.

The investigation revealed that the women had received
pedicures at the same popular nail salon. Samples from the
lesions were sent to the lab and public health inspectors also
took samples of water from the whirlpool footbaths used for the
pedicures. Sure enough, lab tests from the sores and from the
nail salon found traces of *Mycobacterium fortuitum*, an unusual
bug that is commonly found in low levels in the water supply but

rarely causes any problems. In the end, 110 women developed these nasty persistent sores. One young woman's legs had erupted into more than thirty oozing abscesses; another was convinced she had bedbugs and had her entire house sprayed.

*M. fortuitum* had found the perfect conditions to thrive, and it grew to such large numbers that the bug was able to invade any small nicks or cuts in the skin. Women who had shaved their legs in the twenty-four hours before receiving their pedicures had created the perfect entry point for the bug to invade the skin. The boils that result are difficult to treat and sometimes require as much as six months of antibiotics to cure. Even after full-course treatment is completed, most women are left with permanent scars. Improperly cleaned and disinfected whirlpool footbaths set the stage for this outbreak, which left more than a hundred people disfigured.

❋

IN THIS CHAPTER we'll take a walk through the neighbourhood and visit the places where bugs commonly hide. We'll look more closely at salons and spas, public facilities and gathering places, and even our own homes and gardens, and investigate the unusual bugs that sometimes thrive in these environments. We will look at how the divisions of Microbes Inc. have adapted to these locations and what measures we can take to make sure they don't get the upper hand.

## THE GREAT INDOORS

Starting with the many indoor places we visit, let's take a closer look at the impact of Microbes Inc. on our health-care systems and how the superbug phenomenon has spread from hospitals into the rest of the community.

## The Hospital Paradox

Some of the newest and most severe infections have developed in the very places meant to cure illness: our health-care system. The combination of vulnerable patients, crowding, and antibiotic use and misuse has made hospitals a perfect environment for the emergence of new strains of bacteria that are particularly difficult to treat. These superbugs have caused untold suffering in patients already weakened by fighting other illnesses.

Almost as soon as antibiotics were developed in the 1940s, the bugs they targeted began developing ways to get around the medication's killing agent. Within a few short years most strains of bacteria had overcome penicillin, and this pattern has continued for every new drug that has since been developed. The widespread use and, in too many cases, misuse of antibiotics to treat infections, especially viral infections, and the vast amounts of antibiotics used as growth stimulators for livestock have compounded the bacteria's evolutionary will to survive. Nowhere has this effect been more apparent than in hospitals, a setting that offers seemingly endless opportunities for bugs to thrive.

Hospital procedures provide many inviting ways for bugs to invade the human body, from surgical incisions to intravenous lines, catheters, and ventilators. In addition, shared hospital rooms mean shared colonies of bugs. All manner of disease and infection can transfer easily both between patients and between health-care workers and patients, thus allowing the members of Microbes Inc. unique opportunities to mix and mingle and for superbugs to evolve.

*The Super Two:* MRSA *and* VRE

Methicillin-resistant *Staphylococcus aureus* (MRSA) is a super-bug that has developed resistance to several classes of antibiotics; it is characterized specifically for its resistance to the antibiotic methicillin. *Staph aureus* is a bacterium that lives on the human skin and is part of our normal flora. But occasionally when immune defences are down, the bacterium can cause infections of the skin, joints, heart, and lungs, and sometimes more serious, even deadly infections can develop in the blood. The antibiotic-resistant strains of this bacterium are much more difficult to treat, and for many the only antibiotic that works to cure infection is a costly medication called vancomycin, which can be administered only through an intravenous line.

The other superbug that is of great concern is vancomycin-resistant *Enterococci* (VRE), a rare group of bugs that is found almost exclusively in hospitals, causing intestinal infections in unsuspecting patients. These bugs have evolved to become resistant to almost all antibiotics that are currently available, but so far they have thankfully been uncommon. The most frightening prospect for public health officials is that one day VRE and MRSA may exchange bits of genetic material, thus creating a supreme superbug resistant to all antibiotics known.

In October 2007 *Scientific American* published an article on health-care–associated infections under the ominous but telling title "Superbugs and Hospitals: Go in Sick...Get Sicker." The U.S. CDC estimates that 1.7 million people fall ill and 100,000 people die every year from infections contracted at hospitals at a cost of more than US$30 billion. About 95,000 of these health-care–associated infections and

20,000 deaths are caused by MRSA. In Canada, estimates show that a quarter of a million people suffer from health-care–associated infections and over eight thousand people die from these illnesses every year at a cost of CAN$281 million. Sadly, most of these infections are preventable.

MRSA was first detected in hospitals in the United States in 1974 but was not thought at the time to be of particular concern. That same year a study showed that MRSA was the cause of about 2 percent of hospital infections; by 1995 this number had spiked dramatically to 22 percent. How had this happened? For almost twenty years MRSA had gone unchecked in hospitals because of a lack of formal infection-control programs. Health-care workers, like many scientists, were under the impression that antibiotics could prevent and cure all infections. As more and more patients were found to have contracted new forms of disease during their hospital stay, this myth was slowly dispelled. But it took the HIV epidemic during the mid-1980s to renew commitment to infection-control programs in hospitals in a measure to protect both staff and patients.

Governments in Canada and the United States are just waking up to the terrible impact of hospital infections, but other countries have tackled superbugs such as MRSA and come up victorious. In the late 1960s MRSA caused 33 percent of hospital infections in Denmark. In response to these high numbers, health officials established a stringent infection-control program. Patients were tested for the bug when they were admitted to the hospital and were isolated for treatment of MRSA. Strict adherence to handwashing saw infection rates drop dramatically. For the past twenty years hospitals in Denmark have consistently reported less than 1 percent of infections as MRSA.

And Denmark is not alone. The Netherlands and other countries in Scandinavia also reported high rates of MRSA in the 1970s. They used a similar "search-and-destroy" strategy, and the rates have since dropped to 1 to 3 percent of infections. The battle against health-care–associated infections can be won, but requires strong leadership by hospital administrators, governments, and public health networks to combat these ever-changing bugs. What these successes in Europe have taught us is that the most important measure to prevent transmission of disease is for health-care workers, patients, and visitors to clean their hands between each contact. While it may seem shocking, studies show that nurses, doctors, and technicians clean their hands less than 40 percent of the times they should between touching patients. There are many reasons for this: overworked, under-resourced staff; hospital crowding; lack of handwashing facilities. The end result is continued suffering of patients and sometimes of health-care workers who themselves become infected with these new bugs.

In addition, many prevention programs became the victim of their own success. As health care became more expensive and hospitals were forced to look closely at where the money was being spent, infection-control programs became the easy target of budget cuts, since during the 1940s, with the advent of antibiotic treatment, it came to be believed that infections were no longer a threat to human health. But the emergence of new infections such as SARS and the rising number of MRSA and VRE cases in the past few years have finally put these critical programs back on the priority list.

The overuse and misuse of antibiotics is another contributing factor in the emergence and spread of superbugs. Antibiotics work only for infections caused by bacteria and should not be prescribed for viral infections. Most coughs, sore throats, ear infections, and all colds and flus are caused by viruses; antibiotics won't work on these infections and can lead to antibiotic-resistant strains of disease.

While MRSA and VRE are difficult to treat, they can be killed in the environment and on our hands by standard household or hospital cleaning solutions, as well as by plain soap and water and alcohol-based hand rubs. Hospital hygiene is also a key measure that can kill bugs on surfaces and medical equipment. VRE, for example, is known to contaminate the environment, and it can last on bedrails, toilets, or other surfaces for days if they are not properly cleaned. Hospital housekeeping staff can act as key partners in safety by ensuring these bugs are killed by regular and thorough cleaning. While these measures won't solve all the issues around infections in hospitals, they can go a long way in preventing the spread of disease.

*Superbugs Escape*

While MRSA is still most prevalent in health-care settings, in recent years there has been unsettling evidence of outbreaks in people who have not had contact with hospitals. In 1999 a group of children in Minnesota and North Dakota contracted a new strain of MRSA, which resulted in four fatalities. When disease detectives looked into the cluster of cases, they found that a whole new bug had emerged that had some of the characteristics of the hospital MRSA. But this strain had also acquired a piece of DNA that produced a toxin that allowed the bacteria to more easily invade the protective barrier of the skin.

Most *Staph aureus* infections cause common skin conditions such as pimples and small boils. But this new, virulent form of MRSA causes much more severe disease, producing nasty abscesses that are difficult to treat and often require a doctor to drain the infection surgically. In rare cases the bacterium invades the lungs, rapidly dissolving lung tissue and causing an internal flesh-eating disease that quickly leads to death. Public health officials named this new super-bug community-associated MRSA (CA-MRSA) to distinguish it from the hospital-specific bacterial strain.

From military recruits to prisoners, sports teams, injection drug users, homeless people, and even Alaskan natives and First Nations communities, CA-MRSA has been detected where crowding, lack of cleanliness, and shared equipment and personal items such as razors or towels are common. In 2003 nasty skin abscesses from CA-MRSA erupted in players on the professional football team the St. Louis Rams. The infection was traced back to players with "turf burn," skin abrasions acquired from skidding across artificial playing surfaces. The athletes often left these wounds uncovered, leaving them susceptible to contracting disease while roughhousing in the locker room and sharing whirlpool baths, towels, and weights in the training room. The National Football League worked with public health officials to develop standards for cleaning equipment, towel use, and hand hygiene to prevent any future spread of infection. Along with these basic hygiene measures they emphasized the need to cover up cuts and abrasions such as turf burn so that wounds would not become infected. But this bug is not unique to football. CA-MRSA has caused infections in athletes from a variety of sports, especially contact sports such as rugby and wrestling, but soccer, fencing, and even canoeing teams have also been affected.

Like its hospital cousin, CA-MRSA is easily killed on surfaces by using regular cleaning products, and transmission can be prevented through regular handwashing. In addition, it's important to keep cuts and scrapes covered with clean dressings. Avoid sharing towels and personal items like razors, put a barrier such as a towel between yourself and shared equipment in the gym, and make sure the equipment is cleaned regularly. CA-MRSA is spreading rapidly across North America and Europe, and in some places is now the most common cause of skin infections. The CDC estimates that twelve million patients in the United States visit their doctor for skin infections every year, and in some places more than half are caused by CA-MRSA.

While the term "superbug" tends to elicit fear in most people, only in rare cases do MRSA and CA-MRSA cause severe, untreatable infections. Knowing how the bug is transmitted between people and that the best defence is to follow a few simple hygiene rules gives us the tools we need to combat both the fear and the bug itself. In the end, even superbugs are helpless against good hygiene.

*Lurking Spores*

Another dangerous bug that is specific to health-care facilities in the past decade is *Clostridium difficile*, a bacterium whose survival advantage is its ability to form into a hardy spore that is resistant to drying, heat, and even many cleaning agents. These bugs can live happily in a hospital environment for many days or even weeks unless properly cleaned.

C. diff, as it is called in the medical community, is often included in the superbug group, though technically resistance to antibiotics is not the problem with this bug. Rather, it is the bacterium's ability to transfer easily from person to person and last in the environment that makes it so dangerous. C. diff lives quietly in the intestines of as many as 2 to 10 percent of the population without causing illness. But when someone takes antibiotics, these medications can kill the normal bacteria in the gut, allowing these microbes to rapidly expand their territory. As C. diff flourishes it releases a toxin that causes severe diarrhea, and in some people it can lead to a condition called pseudomembranous colitis, which almost always requires the removal of the bowel to cure.

Although C. diff has been documented in patients as far back as 1935, its relationship to diarrheal illness wasn't established until 1978. C. diff has caused outbreaks of diarrhea in hospitals for decades, but for a long time the bacterium was not identified as the cause of the condition because most medical experts thought the bug was part of the normal flora in the gut. It was a series of severe outbreaks in hospitals in Montreal in 2003, and later in Calgary, Ottawa, and other parts of North America, that brought C. diff to the medical community's attention. Public health officials discovered that the bug had evolved to produce excessive amounts of toxin, leading to severe disease in almost all who were affected. Patients who contracted the infection suffered from more copious diarrhea, and the spores were found in much higher numbers in the hospital environment. The more spores, the more bugs, and the greater the chance of passing the disease on to another vulnerable patient.

In 2003–04 more than 7,000 patients in Quebec became ill with C. diff; 1,400 contracted the disease in a three-month period alone, and more than 200 died as a result. The Quebec Ministry of Health soon after announced a $20 million plan to improve infection prevention and control programs in its hospitals, which led to dramatic reductions in C. diff rates, so much so that they are now some of the lowest in the country. Since then C. diff outbreaks have been recorded in hospitals

across Canada and the United States, and a high-profile outbreak in the Maidstone and Tunbridge Wells National Health
Service Trust in England led to the deaths of more than
ninety people. Senior administrators of the trust were
charged in court for failing to implement recommended
infection-control measures to stop the outbreak.

Once again we know how this disease is transmitted and
we know what needs to be done to prevent it. It takes leadership and commitment to improving the infection-control
measures in hospitals, from handwashing to environmental
hygiene. Ideally every person admitted to a hospital would be
offered a single room with its own toilet and sink; this would
not only result in better treatment of patients but would also
protect them from inadvertently picking up someone else's
bugs. In some ways it is hard to believe that we place the most
vulnerable people in hospital rooms with three or four others
who may also suffer from contagious disease, and even ask
them to share a washroom. While it is unlikely that all the
existing hospitals can be converted to single-room facilities, it
is something we should advocate for — for our own protection and for the protection of those we love. In the end,
evidence shows that this measure would cost the health-care
system less money in the long run.

## Public Buildings

Hospitals are not the only places in our community where we
have seen the emergence of new strains of microbes. Any
place where people congregate or where we have developed
systems to regulate the environment, such as air-conditioning
and heating systems, is vulnerable to the many divisions of
Microbes Inc. One famous example of a bug that's found its

home in our modern urban environment is the bacterium *Legionella*. This fascinating microbe burst onto the scene in July 1976, at a convention of American Legion and U.S. military veterans in Philadelphia, Pennsylvania. Hundreds of legionnaires had gathered to celebrate the American bicentennial, and most were staying at the Bellevue Stratford Hotel in downtown Philadelphia. Within days people started to develop pneumonia, and by the time the convention was over 221 people had sought medical care and thirty-four had died.

The U.S. Centers for Disease Control in Atlanta, Georgia, sent a team of epidemiologists to investigate what they feared might be the harbinger of a dreaded influenza pandemic. It took months of intense investigation before disease detectives finally found the microbe that was causing this terrible illness. On January 18, 1977, the CDC announced the newly discovered bacteria, which they named *Legionella* after the veterans who were overwhelmingly affected by the infection.

We have since come to realize that *Legionella* is a hardy bacterium that makes its home in urban water systems. The original outbreak was traced to bacteria growing in the hotel's cooling tower, which was working overtime during the summer convention. Since 1977 *Legionella* has been found to be the cause of hundreds of outbreaks of illness around the world. In 2005 the European Working Group for Legionella Infections reported that more than thirty-two thousand people had become ill with legionellosis in more than six hundred reported outbreaks from 1995–2005 — and those are the ones we know about. Most sporadic cases of *Legionella* go unreported or aren't investigated.

Some of the biggest *Legionella* outbreaks have occurred in locations we might never think would be at risk. In 1989 an outbreak in Louisiana caused illness in thirty-three people ranging in age from thirty-six to eighty-eight; it was traced back to a produce-misting machine at the local grocery store. In 1999 more than two hundred people became ill and at least thirty-two died from legionnaires' disease after attending a flower show in Bovenkarspel, Netherlands; this outbreak was linked to a heated ornamental fountain. Then in 2001 the largest outbreak ever to be reported infected more than eight hundred people in Spain. After much detective work, local public health authorities eventually traced the bacterium to a hospital cooling tower that was releasing clouds of the bugs into the air.

Not everybody is equally at risk of getting sick with *Legionella*. Most of us have robust immune systems that can fight off the bug, as long as we don't inhale too many microorganisms. It is the elderly and those who smoke or suffer from conditions such as lung or heart disease or diabetes who are most susceptible. In 2005, for example, residents and staff at a nursing home in Toronto started falling ill with severe pneumonia. Fear gripped the health-care system, as people worried that this outbreak was a resurgence of the deadly SARS virus. In the end sixty-seven residents became ill, resulting in twenty-seven fatalities — caused by *Legionella*, not SARS. Thirty staff members, twenty-six visitors, and four people who lived or worked in the area also became ill. Eventually the outbreak was traced to the home's cooling tower, which had an overgrowth of the bacteria; it was situated on the roof of the building, next to the fresh-air intake.

*Legionella* loves warm, stagnant water, and the conditions that led to this outbreak were ideal. The air-conditioning system had been working overtime during the summer but had been shut down in early September when the weather started to cool off. When the air-conditioning was turned on again in late September during an unseasonable hot spell, the bugs had a perfect chance to grow. The caretakers would normally clean out the cooling tower at the start of every season, but in this case the system was restarted without first being disinfected — with deadly results. Since this outbreak the regulations for cleaning and situating air conditioners have been revised, particularly for hospitals and long-term care facilities. But *Legionella* outbreaks continue to occur, as this bug has adapted to all sorts of urban devices, including showers, misters, and whirlpools; any warm water environment will do.

### Pedicures, Piercings, and Tattoo Parlours

Another warm water environment that provides perfect conditions for some of the bugs at Microbes Inc. are what are known as personal service settings: nail salons, hairdressers, barbershops, spas, acupuncturists, and body piercing and tattoo parlours. Traditionally these services have not been of great concern to public health officials. However, recent inspections of nail salons and spas, triggered by the outbreak in California in 2000, have revealed that pedicures are far from the only infectious risk posed by these settings. With reuse of unsterilized equipment to cut nails or shave calluses, unclean hand and footbaths, and contaminated wax, the plucking, trimming, and painting that goes on in salons has created an ideal environment for many bugs to thrive.

In San Jose, California, 140 men and women became infected with *Mycobacterium chelonae* (a microbial cousin to *M. fortuitum*) after receiving pedicures in thirty-four different salons in 2004, and similar outbreaks have been recorded in Illinois, Colorado, Washington State, and Oregon. In 2007 a woman in California, who was undergoing cancer treatment, developed an infection caused by an antibiotic-resistant strain of *Staphylococcus* after being given a pedicure, and she died as a result. In Toronto, more than thirty women developed terrible abscesses on their legs, arms, and bodies after receiving acupuncture from needles contaminated with another nasty bug, *Mycobacterium abscessus*. Licensing bodies in many U.S. states and provinces of Canada have now developed standards for cleanliness and disinfection at nail salons, spas, and other personal service settings to reduce the risk of infections. But in a high-volume business these regulations may not be followed as strictly as they should be.

Tattoo and body piercing parlours have also been linked with infections, though for many years these practices were well out of the mainstream, so little attention was paid to these services. In the 1960s tattooing moved beyond the realm of sailors and convicts, and body piercing became trendy in the 1970s after a piercer in California published a magazine called *Body Art*. While facial piercings have long been traditional to many cultures, other body piercings, particularly of the nipples and genitals, are largely a new, Western phenomenon that became popular through the myths propagated by *Body Art*. One of the magazine's most infamous stories suggested that Prince Albert, Queen Victoria's husband and great love, wore a penis ring to avoid unsightly bulges; this story gave birth to a piercing called the "Prince Albert," which enjoyed incredible popularity. Despite its persistence in urban mythology this is undoubtedly an invented story.

Some of the more serious infections that have been linked to tattooing and body piercings are hepatitis B and C. These viruses cause inflammation of the liver and can lead to liver failure, liver cancer, and sometimes even death. Hepatitis B and C are passed from person to person through exchange of contaminated body fluid such as blood, tears, or saliva; hepatitis B can also be transmitted through sexual contact. Over the past decades, tattooing with unclean needles or contaminated ink pots has caused hundreds of people to develop these lifelong infections. Only a minuscule amount of contaminated blood is needed to transmit the infection, but despite the fact that this knowledge has been around for decades, outbreaks continue to be reported. In 2004 a group of people in Toronto contracted hepatitis B after getting tattoos from a temporary stall at a Saturday flea market.

Tattooing and body piercing have also been the cause of other, less lethal but serious infections such as herpes, MRSA, tuberculosis skin infections, fungal infections of the bone, and infections from a virus that causes warts. There have even been rare but concerning reports of infections from dirty tattoo needles that caused blood poisoning, infections of the heart, and even death.

Outbreaks of disease in our neighbourhoods remind us that the divisions of Microbes Inc. are all around us, and we must take the necessary precautions to ensure we are best protected. First, get services only from places that look clean and have a licence. Unlicensed businesses may not follow hygiene regulations, and temporary shops and stalls are unlikely to have adequate facilities to ensure that proper sanitation is maintained.

If you are going for a pedicure, check that the footbaths can be emptied easily and are cleaned between each use. Avoid whirlpool baths, which simply recirculate water and are much more difficult to clean. Ensure that your technician uses sterile equipment when he or she is trimming your nails, and avoid having calluses removed with a razor — a file is much safer. Don't shave or wax your legs twenty-four hours before a pedicure or, if you are having both services done at the same time, ask for the pedicure first.

If you have a medical condition such as diabetes or a weakened immune system, you need to be extra careful about making sure you don't have any scrapes or cuts before going in for one of these services, and that all of the equipment being used is sterile. In fact, it may be better to avoid nail salons altogether. And of course make sure the staff clean their hands regularly (either with alcohol-based hand rubs or soap and water) and especially between each client they work on. And don't be shy about asking the staff about their environmental sanitation procedures; if they don't want to talk about it, you should think about going somewhere else.

If you are going for a tattoo or body piercing, all of the above apply, and be sure to talk with the technician about using disposable ink pots and needles and sterilizing equipment and jewellery. Finally, make sure the jewellery is clean and of good quality and is well positioned, because any kind of skin irritation could lead to infection.

## THE GREAT OUTDOORS

Now that we have looked at some of the indoor environments where bugs have been known to flourish or new strains have emerged, let's consider some of the outdoor spaces where the divisions of Microbes Inc. have also made their home. From pools to parks to our own gardens and backyards, there are many locations in the great outdoors that we should be aware of. Some of these bugs are relative newcomers and others have been in our environment forever. We will look at a few of the microbes that have become part of our surroundings and explore the measures we can take to keep them at bay.

## From the Nile to North America

One emerging newcomer to North America is the dangerous and sometimes deadly West Nile virus. In 1937 the virus was first isolated in a woman suffering from fever in the West Nile region of Uganda. People in the area were becoming ill with fever, headaches, weakness, and muscle aches, and in some cases were developing severe symptoms of encephalitis (infection of the brain) or meningitis (infection of the lining of the brain). While most people had milder disease and recovered after several weeks, the severe form of West Nile virus infection could leave people with long-lasting paralysis and sometimes led to death.

When genetic testing became available several decades later, West Nile virus was found to have been around for as long as a thousand years, causing illness mostly in birds, before the 1937 discovery of the bug in humans. Some historians have even attributed the untimely death of Alexander the Great to the infection because of reports of massive die-offs of birds around the same time. Once the virus was identified, studies showed that the disease was widespread in much of Africa, then spread in Egypt in 1942 and India in the 1950s.

It was in Egypt that scientists were able to tease out the life cycle of the virus and determine how it spread. They discovered that the virus lived and reproduced in the gut of the mosquito, which then transmitted it to people when the insect injected its victim with infected saliva. Several species of mosquito play host to the West Nile virus, and most of them carry the disease after feeding on birds. The West Nile virus multiplies in the bird's blood, although some species are sensitive to the effects of the virus and can die from the infection. Corvids, the family of birds that includes crows, jays, magpies, and ravens, are particularly susceptible to the disease and die in large numbers when the virus is active. The death of crows in particular is an early warning sign that the virus has moved into a new area.

Humans and animals such as horses are only incidentally infected by West Nile, usually when mosquitoes can't find a bird to feed on. There have been outbreaks in human populations in Africa and Israel, as well as countries in Europe. The first large and particularly severe outbreak in Europe was reported in Romania in 1996, when 393 people became ill with West Nile virus infections; 352 of them developed encephalitis and seventeen died. In retrospect this virus has been causing disease in much of Africa, the Middle East, western Asia, and the Mediterranean region of Europe for many decades. But the bug was first reported only in North America only in 1999.

The story of how West Nile virus came to North America is a bit of a mystery, but scientists surmise that the bug probably hitched a ride in an infected mosquito or bird that got onto an airplane from Israel to New York City. In early 1999 genetic testing on the virus in New York proved it was the same bug that was causing outbreaks of disease in Israel. Once the virus reached New York it found a perfect host in the *Culex* species of mosquitoes that were abundant in the city. At first the infections went unnoticed until an astute physician realized that an unusual number of people with meningitis and encephalitis had been admitted to his hospital in the late summer. While he didn't consider that West

Nile virus could be the cause of these diseases, he was worried about other viruses that could cause similar illnesses such as eastern equine and St. Louis encephalitis, which are also transmitted by mosquitoes and had, albeit rarely, caused outbreaks in the city before. He contacted the New York City Department of Health to see if other cases of encephalitis had been reported in the area.

Public health officials launched an investigation that eventually led to the identification of this new arrival. One of the more interesting pieces of the puzzle came from the Bronx Zoo, where veterinarians reported that many of the exotic birds (particularly flamingos) were dying from a severe sickness they had never seen before. Epidemiologists from the CDC were sent to New York City, and after several weeks of intense investigation and a plethora of laboratory tests, West Nile virus, previously unseen in the western hemisphere, was identified as the cause of both the human infections and the illness in the exotic birds. In total fifty-nine people in New York City had become ill with the virus and seven people died, including a Canadian man who was visiting the area in late summer.

The dead flamingos at the Bronx Zoo were a harbinger of things to come. West Nile virus soon spread to birds in neighbouring states, and within three months tens of thousands of birds, mostly crows, had succumbed to the disease. With the approach of colder temperatures in the fall the mosquito vectors became dormant and scientists were left with a big question. Would this virus, never before seen in such cold areas of the world, and certainly never before seen in North America, be able to survive the winter and spread?

Over the winter of 1999–2000 blood samples were taken from residents of the city to try to determine just how many people had been affected by this new virus. Results showed that about 2.6 percent of the population had been infected, which translates to about 8,200 people. The majority were able to fight off the disease and didn't get sick. In addition, their immune systems had now developed antibodies against the virus, which would protect them from future infection. About 1,700 people did suffer from mild illness but thankfully weren't sick enough to seek medical attention; they too had developed antibodies and were now protected. The fifty-nine people who were sent to hospital were mostly over fifty years old, and most had other illnesses such as diabetes or heart disease that made them more vulnerable to severe infection.

After the summer of 1999 public health officials had a pretty good sense of the impact of West Nile virus: most of those who are infected don't get sick at all and about 20 percent develop mild disease. Less than 1 percent — somewhere around one in 150 people — go on to develop the severe form of West Nile virus infection, which causes encephalitis, meningitis, or paralysis. Armed with that knowledge, public health officials across North America waited and watched for what was going to happen next. By the spring of 2000 it became apparent that the virus had survived the winter and was here to stay.

Summer infections in birds and humans were reported in most of the eastern states and along the border with Canada. From there the virus swept across the continent, and by 2007 it had caused disease in all of the contiguous United States and every province in Canada with the exception of British Columbia in the far west. The bug was later also found to be transmitted through organ donations and blood transfusions, and could even be passed from mother to child during pregnancy. We also discovered that we humans are not the only ones vulnerable to the disease: West Nile virus causes illness and death in a wide variety of animals, from domesticated cats, dogs, horses, cattle, sheep, goats, llamas, and alpacas to wild animals such as polar bears, deer, wolves, squirrels, skunks, rabbits, and bats. In addition, the virus was responsible for killing a flock of penguins at the Milwaukee Zoo in 2002 and it decimated an alligator farm in Florida in 2004. The New York City Department of Health reported that the total numbers of West Nile virus–positive specimens in the year 2000 included 1,263 dead birds, four hundred mosquito pools, ten live wild birds, eight sentinel chickens, two bats, twenty-eight horses, one domestic rabbit, one squirrel, one chipmunk, and fourteen humans.

In the years since its arrival in 1999, thousands of people in Canada and the United States have contracted West Nile virus infections, and hundreds have died or suffered long-lasting effects. It has become the most important mosquito-borne disease in North America in just a few short years. It has been a long time since mosquito-borne diseases were a concern on this continent, and many people have never thought about protecting themselves against these outdoor pests. But there are a few precautions we can take around our homes and neighbourhoods to reduce the impact of this new virus on our health.

First, make sure to get rid of any mosquito breeding areas around your house. Mosquitoes need water to breed, so tip over flowerpots and watering cans, drain pools and pool covers, and make sure the water in your pool is changed every few days. It's also important to keep grass short so rainwater doesn't collect on your lawn; even a few tablespoons of water can create an ideal breeding ground for these insects. If you are in an area where there are a lot of mosquitoes, wear a repellent that contains DEET or lemon eucalyptus oil (repellents don't kill mosquitoes but they do make you much less attractive to bite). If you are outdoors in the evening or early morning, when mosquitoes that carry West Nile virus are most active, be sure to wear a long-sleeved shirt and full-length pants, preferably in a light colour, since mosquitoes are more attracted to dark colours.

In most temperate areas mosquitoes are active only in the warmer summer months, although in some areas of the southern United States and Europe they can be active all year round. But we should always keep in mind that in most cases, as long as we make sure to take the necessary precautions to protect ourselves against infection, there is no reason why we cannot enjoy the health benefits and pleasure to be derived from the great outdoors.

## Hot Tubs, Pools, and Water Parks

Other outdoor venues that have emerged in recent years as microbe havens are recreational waters. From backyard hot tubs to local swimming pools, a steady list of bugs has rapidly adapted to thrive in these new environments. In 2003 and 2004 alone, the U.S. CDC reported sixty-two outbreaks of disease from recreational water sources in twenty-six states. Around 70 percent of these cases were reported in treated water sources such as swimming pools and wading pools, while the other 30 percent were in fresh water pools and swimming areas. From these outbreaks almost three thousand people became ill. In about 30 percent of cases, illness was caused by bacteria, with *Shigella* leading the pack; about 25 percent were caused by parasites with *Cryptosporidium* and

*Giardia* being the most common culprits of disease; and about 10 percent were caused by viruses, the majority of which by our ubiquitous friend Norovirus.

Hot tubs became popular in North America in the 1980s when smaller, more affordable models were developed that could be installed on decks or in backyards for personal use. Along with the popularity of hot tubs came a spike in unusual skin infections that were eventually traced back to a bacterium called *Pseudomonas aeruginosa*. These skin infections became so common that they were later dubbed "hot tub folliculitis" by doctors, for the bug's tendency to infect hair follicles. We now know that the bacterium can also be found in large numbers in contaminated whirlpools, on water slides, and even in equipment such as loofah sponges at spas. Most times the skin infection clears up on its own, but the condition can be quite irritating and sometimes requires antibiotic treatment.

*Pseudomonas* is another quirky bug that loves hot water, and it can grow rapidly if water sources are not cleaned, disinfected, and filtered regularly. The water in hot tubs in particular needs to be monitored more closely because the heat breaks down cleaning agents like chlorine faster than in other pools. If you use the communal hot tub at your local gym, make sure it is cleaned regularly and that the disinfectant levels are checked several times a day. It is probably safer to use a large communal hot tub early in the day, since debris such as bits of dead skin builds up with use, and bugs prefer this murky environment.

Along with skin infections, outbreaks of disease caused by the nasty stomach bug *Shigella* have hit unsuspecting recreational water users, both waders and swimmers. This bacterium can cause severe abdominal cramps, nausea, and bloody diarrhea, and as few as ten tiny microbes are enough to make someone sick. In 2001 the first large *Shigella* outbreak was reported at a popular outdoor wading pool at Eagle Point Park in Iowa. Over 150 people, mostly young children, became ill with the same strain of the bacterium *Shigella sonnei*. The pool, in use for more than sixty years, was filled every morning, then drained and cleaned each evening; during the day the water was recirculated through a fountain in the centre of the wading pool.

At some point in early September 2001, one of the many toddlers who frequented the pool leaked diarrhea into the water. The child was infected with *Shigella*, and the bacteria were able to grow and thrive in the pool for several days. If the water had been monitored more carefully the incident might have been averted, but because of the wading pool's design and because the water was not being tested, the chlorine levels were almost at zero. This outbreak awakened health officials to the risk of disease in these outdoor public settings, and across North America special inspection and monitoring programs were developed to test swimming pools, wading pools, water slides, and swimming areas at lakes and beaches. But inspectors are not always able to detect the risks in time.

One of the bugs that has repeatedly evaded inspectors is the parasite *Cryptosporidium*. *Cryptosporidium* is resistant to the killing effects of chlorine, and it can thrive in swimming pools and water parks if the water is not meticulously monitored. In most people the parasite causes classic diarrheal illness, symptoms of which include watery diarrhea and sometimes cramps accompanied by a low-grade fever. The bug can sometimes cause more serious and even fatal illness in those whose immune systems are weakened. People infected with *crypto* can shed the parasite in their stools for up to two weeks following recovery, and in children this can sometimes last several weeks longer.

*Crypto* has caused outbreaks at water parks across North America. One of the largest occurred in the summer of 2005 at a water park at Seneca Lake State Park in upstate New York, where investigators found that two water storage tanks were contaminated. More than 3,800 people reported symptoms of infection, and in mid-August the offending spray pool was ordered closed for the season. In 2007 another outbreak of crypto at an indoor hotel water park in Minnesota caused illness in 58 of the 116 people who used the facility.

Recreational water outbreaks are not unique to North America. One large outbreak reported in Helsinki, Finland, caused 242 people, mostly young children, to fall ill with gastroenteritis just hours after playing in an outdoor wading pool. In this case the highly contagious Norovirus was to blame. Whether they are caused by bacteria, viruses, or parasites, the common factor in all these outbreaks is that someone suffering from gastrointestinal illness has contaminated the water and spread disease. Other factors that contribute to the spread of illness once it's introduced into the environment include improper cleaning of facilities and insufficient chlorine levels to disinfect the water.

This leads to a few simple safety rules to follow when using recreational water such as swimming pools, wading pools, and water parks. The first one is to avoid these public areas if you have gastrointestinal illness, and don't let young children who have diarrhea go in the water. Diapers are not impervious to water, and small amounts of waste can leak into pools. Take children on regular bathroom breaks to avoid accidents, and of course wash your hands after using the toilet or changing diapers. Showering with soap before entering the pool helps prevent the water from becoming contaminated and reduces the chances for growth of bugs in these public environments. While all of these measures seem like common sense, it's amazing how often basic hygiene and public health etiquette are overlooked or forgotten.

## Exotic Animals and Household Pets

Cohabitating with animals, particularly cats and dogs but also other domestic pets — including rabbits, ferrets, guinea pigs, birds, turtles, snakes, and lizards — has been shown to bring happiness and prolong life, but it also comes with some risk of infections. Statistics from the American Pet Products Manufacturers National Pet Owners Survey showed that in 2007, 44.8 million households in the United States had pet dogs and 38.4 million households owned pet cats, as well as 14.2 million fish, 6.4 million birds, 6 million small animals such as hamsters or gerbils, and 4.8 million pet reptiles. All in all this translates to almost 75 million pet dogs, 89 million pet cats, 142 million fish, 24 million small animal pets (including 4.5 million rabbits, 2 million hamsters, 500,000 ferrets, and about 200,000 gerbils), 16 million pet birds, and 13 million pet reptiles (mostly turtles, but snakes and lizards too). The total amount spent on pets in the United States every year is somewhere around $40.8 billion. But the U.S. is not alone in its pet-loving status; statistics from France and Canada report that over half of households own at least one pet, the majority by far being cats and dogs. It should come as no surprise that all this contact with animals can result in infections, and in some instances it has caused large outbreaks. In the United States it is estimated that contact with pets leads to around four million infections every year, at a cost to the medical system of $300 million.

Some of the most common infections associated with pets derive from the ubiquitous bacterium *Salmonella*. *Salmonella* causes mostly self-limited gastrointestinal illness in humans, but the bug can sometimes lead to more severe illness in infants, young children, the elderly, and those with impaired immune systems. The bacterium is exceedingly common in reptiles; it lives in their intestines and on their skin without causing harm to the animals. As a result turtles have long been recognized as a serious cause of illness, especially in young children. In 1975 the CDC estimated that more than 280,000 salmonella infections were directly related to contact with turtles. Turtles smaller than ten centimetres (four inches) were banned for sale in the U.S. in a measure aimed at reducing the number of infections caused by these reptiles. Large turtles also carry the bug, but because the smaller species are more likely to be considered as pets, they pose a higher risk of infection in young children. Despite the ban, outbreaks of salmonella continue to occur from turtles; in 2007 a multi-state outbreak of *Salmonella paratyphi* spread to eighty people across nineteen states. Twenty-four people were hospitalized, three developed bloodstream infections, and tragically a three-week-old infant died. All of them had contracted the infection after playing with turtles.

Reptiles are not the only pets that carry *Salmonella*. Dogs and cats can also contract the bacterium, and, unlike most reptiles, they can develop similar symptoms of infection to humans, including diarrhea, vomiting, fever, and loss of appetite. Like humans, cats and dogs become ill from ingesting contaminated food, particularly raw meat, which has become trendy in some areas in the past few years. This trend has led to a dramatic increase in salmonella infections and infections from E. coli and *Campylobacter*. Not only can cats and dogs become ill with these bacteria, they can shed them in their stools for a long period of time. Many people have contracted illnesses directly after handling pet waste laced with these disease-causing bugs.

In 1999 an outbreak of salmonella in British Columbia, Alberta, and Washington State was traced back to natural pet treats made from dried pigs' ears. Animal-derived pet treats imported from Texas were linked to a second outbreak in Alberta in 2002, and in 2005 nine people became ill after handling dried raw beef, shrimp, and salmon pet treats from Washington State and British Columbia. Then, in 2007, more than seventy people across nineteen U.S. states became ill from *Salmonella* after handling dry pet food that had been contaminated in a manufacturing plant in Pennsylvania. In all these cases pets became ill as well, though the exact numbers are hard to determine since they were not always reported to public health investigators. What is clear is that people were playing with their pets, handling the food or treats, and then ingesting the bugs themselves. Obviously the most important and simplest way to protect ourselves is to wash our hands after contact with our pets.

While salmonella infections are quite common and can be prevented there have been cases of more unusual outbreaks of disease related to contact with non-traditional household pets, which have been enjoying greater popularity in recent years. Since 1992 the number of exotic pets imported into the United States increased by 75 percent; this number includes more than twenty-nine species of rodents, from giant rats to lemmings, hedgehogs, and 1.3 million reptiles. These numbers reflect exotic animals that are legally imported into the country, but the worldwide illegal trade in exotic animals has been estimated to exceed US$10 billion every year, second only to the illegal trade in arms and drugs. Most of these animals are caught in the wild, and most bypass mandatory health screening that helps ensure they are not incubating illness.

One of the most unusual outbreaks reported in the United States was of a disease caused by monkey pox virus. Between May and June 2003, fifty people in Wisconsin, Illinois, Indiana, and New Jersey came down with nasty skin infections and fevers after coming into contact with sick prairie dogs that had been purchased from exotic pet stores. Monkey pox is a cousin to the deadly smallpox virus and had never before been seen in North America. The virus is known to cause occasional skin infections and fevers in parts of Africa, with one of the largest outbreak affecting 338 people in the Democratic Republic of the Congo in 1996–97. While rare, the virus can be fatal if the body is not able to fight off the infection.

Disease detectives from the CDC were called in to investigate after several young children in a daycare developed infections. They had all played with a prairie dog that a neighbour had brought in for show-and-tell. The investigation revealed that monitoring the importation of exotic pets had fallen through the cracks, and few restrictions had been placed on this burgeoning industry. In this case the prairie dogs had been imported to several areas across the country and later had spent time in a warehouse with imported Gambian giant rats. The rats had been infected with monkey pox and became ill sometime in their travels. The virus then spread to the prairie dogs and several other small animals in the collecting centre before they were distributed to pet stores around the country. The fateful prairie dogs didn't show signs of illness until after they had reached pet stores in the Midwest. The end result was that fifty people (mostly children) developed illness, but thankfully the animals succumbed to the infection before the virus could spread to local rodent populations.

Speedy action by public health officials not only stopped the outbreak but may have averted a catastrophe had this terrible bug been able to spread to animals across North America. The governments of both Canada and the United States have started to look at tightening legislation and increasing inspections of imported pets after this dramatic outbreak. The one thing that became clear in both countries is that there is a patchwork system of laws and regulations around the importation of exotic animals, and no single agency has the authority to limit the importation, sale, or even movement of these creatures within the country.

Animals can carry a wide variety of bugs, some of which make them ill and some that use the animal as a vector to transfer disease to humans. Everything from fungal infections to skin infections like scabies and parasitic infections like toxoplasmosis has been linked to household pets. Some imported animals have even been linked to rabies infections, and in 2004 imported pocket pets (gerbils and hamsters) caused an outbreak of the unusual bacterial infection tularemia that spread through parts of Canada and the United States. Several uncommon infections are also related to pets, including skin infections caused by *Mycobacterium marinum*, or fish tank granuloma, which has been linked to contaminated aquariums, and respiratory infections caused by *Chlamydophila psittaci*. This latter bug causes a type of lung infection called psittacosis, or "parrot fever," which was reported in 935 people in the United States between 1988 and 2003. In all cases the bacterium was contracted from pet birds, mostly parrots, parakeets, and macaws.

While there are some hazards to watch out for when owning a pet, the health benefits from animal contact far outweigh the risk of infection as long as a few simple precautions are taken. The most important measure is to wash your hands and to wash the hands of children after playing with pets, handling their food or treats, and even handling their beds or food bowls. In addition, proper disposal of pet waste is important, a task pregnant women should avoid because of the risk of contracting toxoplasmosis. Wearing disposable gloves when cleaning fish tanks is a simple and effective way to avoid picking up bugs from the water. Make sure pets are vaccinated for common illnesses, especially rabies, and are on a flea-control program. And finally, sick animals should always be assessed and treated by your veterinarian.

### Animal Farms and Petting Zoos

Along with exposure to pets in our homes, contact can be made with animals in a variety of public settings. These areas include zoos, petting zoos, agricultural fairs, and farm visits. Between 1991 and 2005 fifty-five outbreaks of disease were reported to public health authorities in Canada and the United States from animal contact in these public settings.

In 1999 an outbreak of the severe gastrointestinal infection E. coli O157:H7 was linked to contact with miniature goats and sheep in a petting zoo at a fall fair in London, Ontario, and in 2004–05, 173 people became ill with E. coli O157:H7 after coming in contact with animals at petting zoos in North Carolina, Florida, and Arizona. The same bug caused infections in fifty-six children who visited farms in Pennsylvania and Washington; nineteen were hospitalized.

The phenomenon is not unique to North America. One large outbreak in Wales affected sixteen children and one adult following a festival at an open farm; ten were hospitalized and three children developed hemolytic uremic syndrome, in which toxins from the bacterium attack the kidneys. Other illnesses that have been linked to animal exhibits are a who's who of players from Microbes Inc., including *Salmonella*, *Campylobacter*, tuberculosis, rabies, *Giardia*, the sheep virus Orf, tularemia, and the fungal infection ringworm. Of course we need to put these outbreaks, tragic as they are, in perspective. More than fifty thousand people visited the farm in Wales without incident, and it is estimated that ten million people frequent the thousand open farms in England and Wales annually. Millions of people also visit fall fairs, zoos, petting zoos, and animal exhibits every year, and most maintain good health.

Guidelines have been developed for animal exhibit operators in Canada, the United States, and the United Kingdom that stress the importance of environmental cleanliness and providing hand-cleaning facilities for visitors. Most of the reported outbreaks are linked to food, either food that was consumed by people while they were visiting the farm or food that was fed to the animals. Cleaning your hands and your children's hands immediately after leaving the area (even if you haven't touched the animals) is the single most important measure that prevents infections. In addition, it's best to leave soothers, baby bottles, and sippy cups at home, because they can become inadvertently contaminated. It should also be noted that human–animal interaction can be incredibly stressful for the animals and can even increase the chances that they will shed bugs in their feces and into the environment.

So guidelines are provided for farmers and zoo staff to create a calm environment for their keep. Human contact with animals, whether as pets in our homes or in settings like zoos and farms, is part of our society, and it can be rewarding and safe as long as we are careful.

❀

WE HAVE NOW come full circle in our walk through the neighbourhood, visiting a selection of areas where the members of Microbes Inc. commonly lurk. Despite the tremendous advances we have made in both preventing and treating infections, there are still old risks we need to watch for and new ones that emerge every day. Whether in our homes, parks, or public buildings the best defence is to wash your hands and to make sure that others clean their hands too. Knowing what to do to prevent infections from animals, from water, and in our own backyards is a good start to staying healthy at home. Next we'll take a look at how these same simple rules can help keep us safe on our travels abroad.

# SIX

## TRAVEL

## BUGS

"I WOULDN'T EAT THAT," the doctor warned her husband as he sat down with the small box of sweets bought from a street vendor on a hot day in Delhi, India. But he would not be deterred; after all, they were just sweets — what could possibly be wrong with them?

The couple had been travelling for several weeks and had covered half a dozen countries, eating everything from street food to gourmet meals at five-star restaurants. Maybe it was a sense of invincibility derived from a lifetime of worldwide illness-free travel that drew him on, or maybe it was just the overwhelming temptation of a delicate, finely decorated local sweet.

"You are way too cautious," was his defence. "I'll be fine."

Maybe he had forgotten for a moment that she was a doctor who specialized in infectious disease outbreaks and how to prevent getting sick.

"Okay, but don't say I didn't warn you," she cautioned, before taking a picture of him to capture the moment.

Sure enough, three days later he awoke feverish, suffering from terrible abdominal cramps, vomiting, and diarrhea. She nursed him through the worst of it over the next two days, searching for fluids he could keep down and then starting him on toast and rice when he began to show signs of recovery. It was a good week before he was well enough that she had the heart to say, "I told you so!"

❀

EVERY YEAR MORE than fifty million people from industrialized nations journey to the developing world, and as many as 70 percent of them report that they contracted some form of illness during their travels. By far the most common malady encountered is what is known as "traveller's diarrhea," or in Mexico the legendary term "Montezuma's revenge," and in India the more colloquial "Delhi belly." Gastrointestinal illness is most often caused by mild strains of E. coli, the ubiquitous bug that turns on the water-secreting cells of the gut. Around fifty thousand people who travel to high-risk countries come down with traveller's diarrhea every day, which often results in the end of a pleasant vacation or interruption of an important business meeting. Thankfully, the illness caused by these strains of E. coli doesn't usually result in long-term damage or serious disease. Statistics show that only 1 to 5 percent of travellers seek medical attention while on their journeys, about one in a thousand will need medical evacuation, and fewer than one in a hundred thousand will die from illness contracted abroad. Most serious illnesses and deaths in travellers are not from the effects of the world of Microbes Inc. but from other causes such as motor vehicle collisions, heart attacks, and, sadly, violence.

While all travel poses some inherent risk of infection, the risk of contracting severe illness varies depending on the type of travelling one does and where one visits. The business traveller who stays in five-star hotels or the vacationer at a beach-side all-inclusive is quite different from the adventure traveller scaling Mount Everest, the medical missionary in rural Uganda, or the family returning to visit relatives in a remote village in India. While many types of travel and travel risks may overlap, the chances of contracting infectious illness can increase depending on the places you visit and the duration of your stay. So let's look at the different kinds of travellers and the most common health risks associated with each.

TRAVEL FOR BUSINESS AND PLEASURE

Let's start with the business traveller and the vacationer and consider what bugs they may need to be prepared for. Both these groups tend to be short-term travellers who for the most part stay in hotels or resorts, many of which offer clean, modern facilities and follow standard sanitary guidelines. The types of risks these visitors may face are usually quite different from those of long-term travellers, who sometimes live in more rustic conditions. Short-term travellers are most often concerned about adapting to different time zones, dealing with the stress of important meetings with people from cultures quite different from their own, or adjusting to an unfamiliar environment where some locals are looking to take advantage of tourists. Couple these issues with isolation from family and friends and different social norms around food, drink, and even sex, and you get a few pitfalls the savvy short-term traveller needs to avoid to stay out of reach of Microbes Inc.

For the business traveller in particular cultural customs around food and water can pose a major challenge. In many countries socializing with clients is a key part of business relationships, but it can be fraught with danger for the inexperienced traveller. Is it okay to decline that special dish containing raw seafood that was prepared in your honour as a guest? Or the glass of cold tap water during a visit to a factory on a humid day? There is no simple answer to these questions, and even the most cautious travellers have occasionally been caught off guard and paid the price later.

For most short-term travellers, ensuring that routine immunizations are up to date is the most important thing to do before heading abroad. Immunizations are not just for children; they are an important part of a lifelong health program to prevent infectious diseases. The health risks encountered during travel are a good reminder about making sure these immunizations are up to date at every age.

Number one on the list for most adult travellers is tetanus. Tetanus is caused by the bug *Clostridium tetani,* which lives everywhere in the environment, both in Western countries and abroad. Everyone must be immunized to prevent this terrible and deadly disease. The bacterium lives in soil, and produces a toxin that affects the body's muscles and nerves, causing painful spasms of the jaw muscles (its nickname is lockjaw) and eventually leading to paralysis of the breathing muscles and death. A booster shot every ten years will ensure that your immune system is fully primed and ready to attack should a cut or scrape occur while travelling, or even just

gardening in your own backyard. Tetanus is no more dangerous abroad than at home, but the treatment for the disease is
tricky and the antitoxin difficult to come by in some parts of
the world. So it's better to be prepared in advance, since there
is no guarantee that access to medical care will be available
in time.

In addition to tetanus, most countries in the world have
vaccination programs to protect children against diphtheria,
polio, whooping cough, and measles, and most Western
countries also include mumps, rubella, and more recently
hepatitis B and chicken pox. The savvy traveller will ensure
that all of these immunizations are up to date. Even a business traveller staying at the best hotels in sophisticated urban
areas of developing countries can be inadvertently exposed to
measles, and in some parts of the world polio and diphtheria
have made roaring comebacks. Vacationers at the best resorts
are sometimes exposed to hepatitis B, especially if their vacation requires a trip to a local health facility, where equipment
such as needles may not be sterilized. For all travellers the
continuing outbreaks of diphtheria, measles, mumps, and
polio remind us how important our immunizations continue
to be, especially in the face of the disappearing risk of many
diseases in most Western countries. Once at their destination,
however, the most important measure business travellers and
vacationers can take to avoid getting sick is to be obsessive
about good hygiene and careful about food and drink.

## Montezuma's Revenge

The most common illness all travellers suffer from is gastrointestinal upset. Typical business and vacation travellers tend
to take shorter trips and often stay in hotels in sophisticated

urban centres or at high-end resorts. These clean and some-times luxurious environments can give many travellers a false sense of security. Even at five-star hotels in China, Southeast Asia, Africa, and South America, the infrastructure may not be developed enough to ensure that the water is safe to drink. Many hotels have their own filtration plants or promise that the water is boiled before being served to guests, but unless you are absolutely certain these practices are in place it is best to avoid drinking the water. Bottled water has its own risks but for the most part is a safe alternative in most developing coun-tries. While there have been horror stories about restaurants or merchants refilling plastic water bottles with tap water or water from a contaminated stream, these incidents are thank-fully rare and tend to happen in smaller city centres.

Avoiding tap water can be harder than one might imagine, even for the high-end business traveller. For one thing it means using bottled water to brush your teeth and being extra careful not to swallow water while showering. One common mistake that has led to countless days of misery is drinking a beverage with ice cubes. Some bugs that cause the most ser-ious illness — bugs such as the bacterium *Shigella* — can make you sick if you ingest as few as ten microbes — far fewer than you would even notice in a glass of water or an ice cube.

Besides bottled water, other drinks that are widely avail-able and relatively safe to consume are hot drinks such as tea and coffee and cold drinks such as pop and beer. Sticking to these choices is usually a safe bet. Fruit juices are frequently mixed with water, so be cautious about these beverages and don't be afraid to ask hotel staff if water was used to make the juice, and if so whether the water was treated or boiled first. Unpasteurized milk can also be a concern, so always check the label before consuming. This measure is particularly important for young children, the elderly, and people whose immune systems are not at full capacity.

When it comes to food in developing countries, the best advice can be summed up in these few words: "Wash it, peel it, boil it, or forget it." What this saying suggests is that hot foods are generally safe to consume, though you may want to remove the fresh garnish from the plate, depending on where you are eating. It's safest to avoid salads, because it is very difficult to wash them adequately to remove all the offending bugs. Any fruit or vegetable that is peeled is pretty safe, and other produce that can be washed thoroughly in safe water are most often just fine.

## Dangers from the Sea

Raw or undercooked seafood can be a real temptation in many countries, but these foods have been linked to count-less outbreaks of illness caused by everything from viruses such as Norovirus and hepatitis A to bacteria like *Listeria* and even the dreaded cholera. One particularly severe outbreak of Norovirus in 2006 was thought to have infected as many as three million people who consumed the ever-popular raw seafood items sashimi and sushi in Japan. The outbreak so alarmed the Chinese government that it issued a travel advis-ory to its citizens to avoid eating raw seafood in Japan.

Raw seafood is also a staple in many Latin American countries. The traditional dish ceviche, which consists of raw fish marinated in lemon or lime juice, has led to outbreaks in travellers and locals alike. In December 2008 the govern-ment of Chile reported 493 cases of infection from the bacterium *Vibrio parahaemolyticus*; all the cases were linked to the consumption of raw seafood. *Vibrio* is a close cousin to the bug that causes cholera and is commonly found in South American waters during the summer months. The bacterium causes a very unpleasant illness, symptoms of which include nausea, vomiting, diarrhea, headache, and fever, and it can last anywhere from a few days to a week.

Raw seafood has been linked to thousands of cases of illness in Chile over the years; more than eleven thousand cases of gastrointestinal infection were reported in the summer of 2004 alone. There have been outbreaks of cholera in travellers who ate raw seafood in Thailand, and in Hong Kong the illness was linked to contaminated fish tanks in several high-end restaurants. In 1994 a cholera outbreak in Bari, Italy, was traced back to the consumption of raw mussels. All of these incidents prove that there is really no safe place to eat raw seafood. But travellers to developing countries, especially in South Asia, Southeast Asia, and Latin America, where hygiene standards are lower and monitoring programs are non-existent, should be on particular guard.

## Hepatitis A

Another common bug in areas where sanitation is poor is hepatitis A. This virus causes inflammation of the liver, fever, and jaundice. Hepatitis A is most often transmitted through contaminated food or water. The virus is common in many popular vacation spots in Latin America and Southeast Asia but is also known to cause outbreaks in developed countries, most frequently when unwell food handlers pass the virus on to unsuspecting customers who consume the prepared meal.

An outbreak in Toronto at a popular grocery store was caused by an employee who prepared fruit and vegetable plates. The virus is killed rapidly by high heat, but the fruit and vegetable plates were meant to be eaten raw. Several customers fell ill and the local public health department immunized almost twenty thousand people who had eaten fruits and vegetables from the grocery store to prevent them from getting sick too. Another particularly large outbreak in Pittsburgh, Pennsylvania, in 2003 affected almost six hundred people who ate at a local restaurant. In both these cases — and in fact in most outbreaks of hepatitis A in North America and Western Europe — the infections were caused by people who had picked up the bug while travelling and spread the virus to others following their return home. A large outbreak in Germany saw 271 people who stayed at the same hotel in Egypt between June and August 2003 become ill with the virus. An investigation by German public health officials found another fifty-nine people in eight other European countries who had also contracted hepatitis A. They too had been guests at the same hotel in Egypt.

So why don't we see hepatitis A outbreaks in those countries where sanitation systems are poor? Essentially, people who live in those areas are exposed to the virus very early in life and most develop immunity to the disease as adults. Hepatitis A tends to cause much milder illness in children who suffer at most from diarrhea and a few days of malaise, while in adults symptoms such as jaundice, fevers, headaches, abdominal pain, and malaise can last for weeks.

For the vacationer and business traveller, hepatitis A lurks in tap water, ice cubes, salads, and raw seafood, and it takes sometimes up to six weeks before signs of infection manifest. This means that people can pass the virus on to family members at home before they develop symptoms such as the telltale jaundice. An effective vaccine for hepatitis A has been available since the mid-1990s, and travellers to parts of the

world where sewage systems and sanitation are not standard-
ized would be wise to receive immunization before their
voyage. While the vaccine won't protect you from all food-
and water-borne infections, it will save you from a serious
and miserable bout of illness that can drag on for months.

The other key to staying healthy while eating abroad is to
meticulously wash your hands before eating and after using
the toilet. It's a good idea to bring a bottle of alcohol-based
hand sanitizer with you and to keep it handy for those times
when soap and water cannot be found. Cleaning your hands
frequently is the key to ensuring that you don't give the bugs
an easy passage into your gut. These simple rules cover many
but by no means all the scenarios business travellers or vacationers might find themselves in while dining in a foreign
country, but sticking to them will help reduce the chances of
getting a nasty infection. As with all things in life, there are
no guarantees. Even the most experienced travellers have
fallen prey to the covert ways of Microbes Inc.

## Water Bugs

The other issue that vacationers and sometimes an unlucky
business traveller may need to think about is risks in water,
both from swimming and from water sports such as snorkel-
ling, diving, or surfing. As we saw in previous chapters, some
bugs live quite happily in swimming pools, ponds, and even
salt water. In many countries where sanitation systems are
not well developed, raw sewage is dumped directly into rivers
or into the ocean very close to shore. These areas can be
teeming with microbes, including bacteria like *Cholera* and
*Salmonella*, viruses like Norovirus and hepatitis A, and parasites like *Giardia*. While on vacation it is important to stick to

safe swimming areas and to avoid swallowing the water as much as possible.

Cuts and scrapes, especially from coral, can lead to some nasty skin infections. A variety of bugs live in coral, and cuts or scrapes from its sharp edges can become infected. Wearing shoes or sandals in areas with coral or sharp rock is the best defence, and if you do get cut, wash the area with warm water as soon as possible and use an antibiotic ointment to help prevent infection. In fact, it's a good idea to add an antibiotic ointment to the list of things to take with you on vacation, as reliable supplies can be hard to find in some areas of the world.

## Love Bugs

The next issue to consider is the possibility of risky sexual behaviour while travelling. This of course applies at home as well, but the potent combination of loneliness or vacation recklessness, increased alcohol consumption, and different social norms can increase the possibility of sexual contact abroad. In some cultures social activities with business colleagues may routinely involve trips to strip clubs and prostitutes. Not surprisingly, the divisions of Microbes Inc. have exploited this avenue of direct contact to thrive just as well as all the others.

The history of sexually transmitted infections, or STIs, as we now call them, goes back as far as written records; prostitution is often called the oldest profession. STIs have been given many names throughout the ages, but in the past two centuries the common term used was "venereal disease," after the Latin name for Venus, the Roman goddess of love. Even the euphemism "social disease" was once popular.

Over thirty bugs can be transmitted sexually, including bacteria, viruses, and parasites. The World Health Organization estimates that one million people every day contract a sexually transmitted infection. The WHO also estimates that 340 million new cases of treatable STIs (including chlamydia, gonorrhea, and syphilis) are diagnosed every year in people between the ages of fifteen and forty-nine, with the majority being in South and Southeast Asia, followed by sub-Saharan Africa, Latin America, and the Caribbean. Millions of viral infections are also transmitted sexually every year, including HIV, genital herpes, and hepatitis B. These viral infections cannot be cured with any medications that we have today. Let's start our tour of the Love Bugs Division of Microbes Inc. by looking at two of the most successful microbes on the planet, *Chlamydia trachomatis* and *Neisseria gonorrhoeae.*

*Chlamydia: The Silent Disease*
Chlamydia is a sexually transmitted infection of the genital tract caused by the bacterium *Chlamydia trachomatis*, a fussy bug that can survive only by living inside human cells. The bacterium was discovered in 1907 in Berlin by scientists Ludwig Halberstädter and Stanislaus von Prowazek and was named after the Greek word for cloak. Chlamydia is often called "the silent disease" because three-quarters of the women and half of the men who have it don't know they are infected. When symptoms do appear, women tend to have a whitish discharge and experience pain during urination, a symptom shared with men, who may also experience swelling of the testicles.

Despite the advent of effective antibiotic treatment for chlamydia in the 1950s rates of infection continue to rise. The United States alone reported over one million new cases in 2007, and those are only the reported cases. The CDC estimates that 2.8 million people are infected in the United States every year, and rates have been steadily increasing worldwide since the 1960s. The impact of chlamydia infections is hardest on women, who can suffer from pelvic infections, infertility, and a higher risk of ectopic pregnancy. The disease can affect babies born to infected mothers, leading mostly to eye infections in newborns. In most Western countries babies' eyes are treated at birth to prevent the spread of infection, but in many developing countries chlamydia remains an important cause of blindness in children.

*Gonorrhea: The Not-So-Silent Disease*
The history of gonorrhea is even more storied than that of chlamydia. In 1879 the German scientist Albert Neisser discovered the bug that caused the disease, which for years had been mistaken for syphilis. The newly discovered bacterium was named *Neisseria gonorrhoeae* after its founder and the Greek words *gonos* (seed) and *rheein* (to flow). Up until 1937 gonorrhea was untreatable and caused most of its damage in women, who suffered infertility and pelvic infections, and their children, who could develop eye infections and more rarely pneumonia. Most men had few symptoms other than short periods of painful urination, releasing a dramatic greenish discharge. In the Victorian era gonorrhea was said to ruin marriages but not lives.

Once penicillin became available in the 1940s it was used widely to treat gonorrhea, but inevitably bacterial resistance to the antibiotic soon emerged. Medical professionals then began using sulpha drugs to cure the disease until resistance made them obsolete in the 1970s. Gonorrhea has since developed resistance to several other medications, and in many places around the world we are down to a single class of antibiotics that still work to cure the disease.

Gonorrhea is second only to chlamydia in causing large numbers of infections transmitted through sexual contact. In 2007 alone more than 350,000 cases of gonorrhea were reported in the United States. Rates in most Western countries were falling from 1975 until the late 1990s, but there has been an unfortunate resurgence of the disease in the past decade, and most strains are proving increasingly resistant to antibiotics. As with all STIs, in any area where poverty, drugs, and prostitution thrive, so too does gonorrhea.

*Syphilis: The Great Imitator*
The third bug in the bacterial STI triumvirate is *Treponema pallidum* or "pale thread," a delicate corkscrew-shaped bacterium that causes the venereal disease known as syphilis. Syphilis hit Europe like a storm in 1495, affecting the armies of Charles VIII of France during the siege of Naples, Italy. After they had conquered and pillaged the city, reports soon emerged of soldiers suffering from genital sores that progressed to full-body rashes, which then developed into deep ulcers that ate away at the nose, lips, eyes, and genitals, leaving disfiguring scars. Those who contracted the disease suffered from a slow, painful death that could last from months to years, and seemingly no one was immune.

At the dawn of the sixteenth century syphilis was known throughout Europe, from France, Switzerland, and Germany to Denmark, Sweden, Holland, England, Scotland, Greece, Poland, and Russia. The disease was carried to all parts of the world during the age of exploration and colonization; it was considered an occupational hazard for soldiers and sailors. The Portuguese explorer Vasco da Gama and his men introduced the disease to Calcutta in 1498, and by 1520 syphilis had spread to Africa, China, and Japan. Countries around the world took to naming the stigmatizing disease after those they believed had brought it to their shores. So syphilis was "the Italian disease" in France, "the French disease" in Germany and England, "the Spanish disease" in the Netherlands, "the Polish disease" in Russia, "the Russian disease" in Siberia, and "the Chinese disease" in Japan.

It wasn't until the nineteenth century that the term "syphilis" was used to describe the illness. The name arose from a moralistic Latin poem, *"Syphilis sive morbus gallicus"* ("Syphilis or the French Disease"), written in 1546 by the Italian physician and poet Girolamo Fracastoro, who recounted the myth of Syphilus, a shepherd who incurred the wrath of the Greek god Apollo and was punished by being afflicted with "foul sores." This story echoed the common sentiment of the time that venereal diseases were punishment for those who had been blasphemous or immoral. Today we have a far greater knowledge of these diseases and how they are transmitted, but we still run into moralistic preaching about STIs, as the HIV epidemic of the 1980s can attest. Despite the moral concerns surrounding syphilis, the disease affected people of all walks of life, including King Charles VIII, Pope Alexander Borgia, Peter the Great of Russia, and even Ivan the Terrible, whose insanity near the end of his days was attributed to the final stages of the disease.

The other controversy that arose around syphilis was the origin of the disease. Why did syphilis emerge with such force in the late 1400s in Europe? The fifteenth century marked the great age of exploration, and historians point out that this epidemic emerged just after Columbus and his men returned from the New World. There is some evidence that diseases caused by bacteria similar to *Treponema pallidum* were causing illness in the newly discovered Americas — diseases such as yaws and pinta — but no definitive evidence has been found to prove that syphilis originated there. The controversy continues today, but the possibility certainly does exist that this was one of the few diseases, if not the only, that spread from the New World to the Old. Others argue that the bug was likely present in Europe in a milder form for some time, and that the wars and concurrent movements of people to large, crowded cities led to the bacterium's ability to evolve into a more severe form.

The bug itself was discovered in 1905, and for many years the only treatment thought to be effective was a mercury-based drug that poisoned as many people as it cured. Paul Ehrlich developed the first true cure for syphilis in 1910 with his arsenic-based drug salvarsan, although it too had many side effects that made the cure almost as bad as the disease. Finally with the advent of penicillin in the 1940s, syphilis could be cured quickly and safely. In the 1920s more than nine thousand Americans died every year from syphilis and more than sixty thousand babies were born with the congenital form of the disease. With the advent of antibiotic treatment these numbers dropped rapidly in the United States and around the world, reaching their lowest numbers ever in the year 2000. At that time elimination programs were being considered in North America and in some European countries, but unfortunately they were not to be.

Rates of syphilis have since increased, and disease patterns show that it is primarily men who are becoming infected. Changing behaviours around risky sexual contact, especially in gay male communities, and the rise of prostitution for drugs have given syphilis a second chance. More ominously, syphilis infections, along with other STIs such as gonorrhea and herpes, seem to increase the risk of becoming infected with HIV as well.

*Herpes: A Lifelong Disease*
The viruses that cause STIs are in a class of their own, both for the potential severity of the disease they cause and for the fact that they are all incurable, despite many advances in treatment options in the past fifteen years. Herpes simplex virus type II is the most common form of the virus that causes genital herpes. Type I most often causes blister-like sores on the face called cold sores and is not considered an STI, although it can certainly be transmitted by some forms of sexual contact.

Herpes was known as far back as Ancient Greece, when the lesions were described in the writings of Hippocrates. The name *Herpes* is Greek for "to creep" or "to crawl," an apt description of the lesions that slowly appear on the surface of the skin. Genital herpes was first described in 1736 by Jean Astruc, court physician to King Louis XIV, in a paper he published on his surveillance of French prostitutes called *"De Morbis Veneris."* The disease was also thought to be familiar during William Shakespeare's time. In his famous tragedy, *Romeo and Juliet*, the character Mercutio describes the fairy queen: "O'er ladies' lips, who straight on kisses dream, which oft the angry Mab with blisters plague." It wasn't until 1873 that the French physician J. B. Vidal proved that herpes had an infectious cause, and it wasn't until the 1950s that the virus was discovered. Despite dire warnings about genital herpes for the past five decades, the virus remains one of the most common STIs.

The highest rates of herpes infections are in sub-Saharan Africa, where the WHO estimates that as many as 80 percent

of women and 50 percent of men between fourteen and nineteen years of age are infected with the disease, while in Asia
and South America the rates are around 30 to 40 percent and
in the United States about 19 percent. These figures represent
an astounding number of people who suffer recurrent bouts
of the small, painful blisters caused by the virus and who have
the potential to pass the infection on to their sexual partners.
Some antiviral medications can lessen the frequency and
severity of each episode, but they are not commonly available
in the places of the world with the highest burden of disease.
So once again prevention is by far the best option. As the old
adage goes, "Unlike love, herpes is forever."

*HIV and AIDS: A World-Altering Pandemic*
Prevention is also the best defence against HIV (human
immunodeficiency virus), the bug that causes AIDS (acquired
immune deficiency syndrome). This virus burst onto the
international stage in the early 1980s when its devastating
effects on gay male communities in the United States led to
outbreaks of unusual infections such as *Pneumocystis carinii*
pneumonia and Kaposi's sarcoma. Public health officials in
San Francisco were among the first to investigate these clusters of rare illnesses. They came to the conclusion that a new
and deadly bug was attacking the immune systems of men in
the community, leaving them vulnerable to infections most
people could fight off. The term AIDS describes the stage of
the disease when the immune system is no longer able to
stave off infection.

A race between scientists led by Robert Gallo at the U.S.
CDC and medical researchers led by Luc Montagnier at the
Pasteur Institute in Paris soon led to the discovery of the cause
of this devastating disease. In May 1983 the French group

discovered a new virus they thought was causing AIDS. But their work was largely overlooked until the CDC announced their discovery of the virus almost a year later, in April 1984. In a courtroom case that was later dramatized in the Hollywood movie *And the Band Played On*, the French team was able to prove that not only did they discover the virus first but the CDC's results had been derived from samples the Pasteur Institute had sent to them for verification. In 2008 Montagnier won the Nobel Prize in Medicine for his work in HIV research.

In retrospect this new virus, named HIV, had probably been circulating in parts of Africa for several decades. It was found in a look-back study that used an archived blood sample taken from a person from central Africa in 1959. Sometime in the 1970s the bug was introduced into the United States, probably by a traveller to Africa, and found a perfect environment to spread in the sexually promiscuous gay communities of San Francisco and New York. Legend has it that the disease was introduced into the United States by a Canadian flight attendant, labelled "Patient Zero" by the press. Scientists working to trace the origin of the virus had actually labelled the samples from this man "Patient O" for "Out of California." But the facts were misrepresented in a published report and the Patient Zero concept stuck, leading to the vilification of the poor young man. In reality it was almost certainly more than one man who brought the virus to America.

The emergence of HIV and AIDS in North America led to the stigmatization of the gay community that hindered efforts by public health officials to investigate its causes and find treatments. As happened in the fourteenth century with venereal diseases, there was tremendous prejudice against the communities first affected, often with much moralizing and very little compassion. Over time we have come to understand that the global scourge of HIV affects everyone, not just gay men, though efforts in many places to combat this slow-moving pandemic remain feeble and inadequate. But all is not lost.

On World AIDS Day in 2008, Dr. Margaret Chan, Director-General of the WHO, called AIDS "the most devastating infectious disease humanity has had to face." Thankfully, attitudes prevalent at the start of the epidemic have changed; partnerships have been formed among public health officials, the affected communities, religious leaders, and researchers, and treatments have been developed that help contain the disease if not cure it. The challenge now is to provide access to treatment for the millions of people affected worldwide, particularly in low- and middle-income countries.

A search for a vaccine continues, but the HIV bug has proven elusive, rapidly changing to avoid human immune defences and the killing effects of all available medications. In 2007 the WHO estimated that 33.2 million people were living with HIV or AIDS worldwide, with 90 percent of the burden of illness in the sub-Saharan countries of Africa, where it is the leading cause of death. It estimates also that there are 2.5 million new infections every year, which translates to 7,500 newly infected people every day; 2.1 million people die from AIDS annually. In the countries with the highest burden of disease, HIV affects both men and women and is transmitted primarily through sexual contact. In sub-Saharan Africa, a mind-boggling two-thirds of the population is living with HIV.

In other areas of the world the epidemic is concentrated to specific groups: men who have sex with men, injection drug users, and commercial sex workers. For example, in Canada, a country of 37 million people, about 63,000 people are living with HIV or AIDS, and about 2,500 to 4,500 new infections are reported every year. The percentage of women infected rose from 11 percent in 1985 to 27 percent in 2007, and about 40 percent of the women acquired the virus through use of injection drugs. Overall, 51 percent of reported cases are in men who have sex with men, 32 percent are from heterosexual contact, and 17 percent are in injection drug users. The epidemic in the United States shows similar proportions, but what is hidden in these numbers is the effect of drugs, prostitution, and poverty, which are the underlying drivers of the disease in much of the world. The HIV epidemic in South and Southeast Asia is largely associated with commercial sex workers, their partners, their clients, and their clients' partners. HIV brings home the notion that you are exposed to all the former lovers your sexual partner has ever had.

This, in a circuitous way, brings us back to travel. Sexual contact brings risks, of both embarrassing but treatable STIs and ones that can change your life. Travel to certain areas of the world is riskier than others, but engaging the services of prostitutes has inherent dangers everywhere. The business traveller who socializes with clients in a country that makes prostitutes available or the vacationer who is lured by the availability of sex workers in a foreign land should consider ahead of time how he will deal with the risk of sexually transmitted infection. The only sure defence is abstinence, but after that, using condoms is the most effective preventive measure for all STIs. This measure, of course, is not just for the business traveller or vacationer; it applies just as much for any traveller and for those back home.

## Hepatitis B

There is another member of the Virus Division of Microbes Inc. that both business and vacation travellers should think about both before and during their trip abroad: hepatitis B. This bug can be transmitted through sexual contact but also through any kind of contact that exposes a person to infected blood, tears, saliva, or semen. It takes only a minute amount of contaminated fluid to transmit the disease, making it one of the most infectious bugs around.

While the virus itself wasn't discovered until 1965, the disease it causes has been around for much longer. Jaundice was described as far back as Hippocrates, and outbreaks of what we now know as hepatitis B infections were first recorded in the late 1880s. The first detailed recording of an outbreak of jaundice was reported in dock workers in Bremen, Germany, in 1883, and was described by the German researcher A. Lurman in a classic paper in 1885. During that time an ongoing smallpox outbreak was affecting the population of Bremen and almost 1,300 dock workers had been treated with a vaccine made from human lymph. Over the next eight months 191 workers developed what Lurman described as "icteric illness," or jaundice. In what has become a classic epidemiologic study, he showed that all those affected had received their vaccine from a batch of lymph that proved to be the cause of their subsequent illness. Workers who were vaccinated with other batches of lymph remained well. Outbreaks of this jaundice-inducing disease became more common after the invention of the hypodermic needle in 1909. Ironically many of the outbreaks were caused by reusing hypodermic needles to inject the new drug salvarsan to treat syphilis.

By 1947 scientists suspected that this disease of the liver was caused by an infectious agent, most likely a virus, but it was another twenty years before the bug was finally identified by Baruch Blumberg, a scientist with the U.S. National Institutes of Health, while he was researching diseases in Australian Aborigines in 1965. The virus itself was first seen under the electron microscope in 1970, and by the 1980s its genome had been sequenced, which allowed researchers to begin work on a vaccine.

Like the other hepatitis viruses, hepatitis B has a predilection for the liver, where it can cause serious inflammation and in some cases cirrhosis, or scarring, leading to the complete destruction of the liver. It can also cause liver cancer in people who are chronically infected. The liver is essential for clearing the blood of toxins, and when it is not working properly some of these toxins can build up, resulting in the characteristic yellow colouring of the skin known as jaundice. Most people who are infected manage to clear the virus on their own after a few weeks of miserable illness, but about 20 percent of those affected with the disease are never able to rid their body of the bug, which then causes chronic infection that can be passed on to others.

About one-third of the world, or two billion people, have been infected with hepatitis B, and there are about 260 million chronic carriers of the virus. The highest proportion of chronic carriers who can pass the disease on to others is in Asia, Southeast Asia, and Africa. Sexual contact and contaminated needles are the most common ways people contract hepatitis B while travelling.

Using condoms for sexual contact is an important measure to protect against hepatitis B, but by far the best protection is vaccination. An effective and safe vaccine has been available since the mid-1980s but it requires a bit of planning. The vaccine is given in a series of three injections: a first; a second, one month later; and a third, six months after the first. While it takes some time to get full protection against the disease, the protection lasts for life, so it is well worth it. In many countries public health programs immunize all children against hepatitis B, so in time the risk the virus poses should greatly diminish.

## LONG-TERM TRAVELLERS

The next class of traveller is those who journey for longer periods of time and may stay in more rural or remote areas to work or seek adventure. Aid workers, missionaries, and adventure travellers all fall into this category, and their risk of encountering the denizens of Microbes Inc. goes up exponentially over that of the vacationer or business traveller. As the risk of infection goes up, so too should the thought and time devoted to preparing for this kind of travel. The list of immunizations that the long-term traveller should consider also gets longer. Routine immunizations are a must, as the chances of encountering someone with measles, polio, or diphtheria are much greater for someone who is, for example, working at a displaced persons camp or teaching in a remote area.

While it may be an option to consider for the short-term traveller, the person embarking on this type of adventure should have immunity against hepatitis A and B. The many opportunities to become infected with hepatitis A defy even the best attempts to avoid contaminated food and water, and you may not have complete control over what you eat or drink if you are living in a rural community for a long period of time. Immunization against hepatitis B is also essential, particularly if you will be working in any sort of health-care situation or are setting out on an adventure that may lead to accident or injury. Safe needles are a rarity in many parts of the developing world, and hepatitis B is a real risk if an injection is needed. For people embarking on aid work or high-risk activities it may be wise to bring your own sterile needle with you just in case.

The list of immunizations that this type of traveller should have includes routine vaccines such as tetanus, diphtheria, polio, pertussis (whooping cough), measles, mumps, rubella, and hepatitis A and B. In addition, there are a number of immunizations these travellers should consider, depending on where they are going and the time of the year. One important immunization is for protection against yellow fever.

## Yellow Fever

Yellow fever is a disease caused by a virus that is transmitted to humans from mosquitoes. It was named after the characteristic yellowing of the skin and eyes caused by jaundice, which results from liver inflammation. The disease-causing yellow fever virus is found only in Africa and South America, but the mosquito that transmits the virus is much more widespread, so many countries regularly monitor for the disease in case it is introduced into the area by an infected traveller. The disease itself ranges from mild illness with fever and muscle aches to life-threatening illness in which the patient is fraught with fever, chills, muscle and headaches, and vomiting that can lead to shock, bleeding, and kidney and liver failure after several days. An ominous sign of illness is dark urine from the virus's destructive effects on the kidneys.

Yellow fever has been known for more than four hundred years, and was one of the main reasons that colonization attempts by Europeans failed in many areas of Africa. It was also a major factor in the failed attempt by Napoleon to defeat a slave revolt in Haiti in 1802; 22,000 of the 25,000 troops he sent to the island succumbed to the ravages of the disease. During the age of exploration, massive outbreaks erupted in European cities after travellers returned from Africa. In the 1700s epidemics of yellow fever affected hundreds of thousands of people in Italy, France, Spain, and England. During the nineteenth century more than 300,000 people were said to have died from yellow fever in Spain alone. British and American troops died by the thousands in the attempted invasion of Cuba in 1762–63, and a massive outbreak in Philadelphia in 1793 killed as many as 10,000 people.

In 1881 the Cuban scientist Carlos Finlay determined that yellow fever was transmitted by mosquitoes. During that time the miasma theory still reigned, so for decades much of his work was ignored by the medical community. It was Walter Reed, a U.S. Army surgeon, who finally confirmed Finlay's work in the early twentieth century and proposed mosquito-control initiatives to stop the spread of the disease. His recommendations were put to the test during a massive outbreak in New Orleans in 1905. Fumigating houses, covering drinking-water cisterns, and treating pools of standing water with kerosene were some of the methods that were applied to protect people from mosquitoes carrying the disease. Despite initial skepticism, the measures proved successful. Reed's methods were soon adopted in Canada and the United States, and since then there have been no major outbreaks of yellow fever in North America. The effectiveness of Walter Reed's methods led to an attempt by the Rockefeller Foundation in 1913 to eradicate the disease around the world. The complex nature of the mosquito–virus cycle, however, stymied this attempt, and the initiative was eventually abandoned.

The yellow fever virus has two main cycles: one in the urbanized human environment, where the *Aedes* mosquitoes that carry the virus are well established, and the other affecting mainly monkeys living in areas of tropical rainforest. This second cycle, called the sylvatic or jungle variety of yellow fever, is impossible to interrupt with mosquito-control measures because the insects selectively breed in the jungle's tree canopy. Urban yellow fever has for the most part been effectively controlled, but outbreaks still occur in some areas of the world where people such as forestry workers and miners work in or near the jungle environment, then travel back to their urban homes, which become a new reservoir for the disease.

Yellow fever has been tempered by the development of a vaccine in 1937 by Max Theiler, a scientist at the Rockefeller Foundation. This vaccine is highly effective; a single injection confers immunity for at least ten years and probably for much longer. It was widely used for the first time in French West Africa in 1939, and effectively stopped the disease in that area. Some countries in Africa have included the vaccine for yellow fever in their childhood immunization programs, but unfortunately the countries most affected by the disease are often the ones that lack effective public health systems to maintain levels of immunization.

Despite the existence of an effective vaccine, the WHO estimates that every year about 200,000 people become ill with yellow fever and 30,000 people die from the disease. The countries at highest risk include thirty-three countries in Africa that straddle the equator (from 15 degrees north to 10 degrees south), with a combined population of over 500 million people, and nine countries in South America, along with several Caribbean islands. In South America, Bolivia, Brazil, Colombia, Ecuador, and Peru have the highest risk of yellow fever, and periodic outbreaks still affect thousands living in urban areas. Widespread immunization has been effective at controlling outbreaks, but with every outbreak it is too late for those initially infected, including travellers. And because the *Aedes* mosquitoes that carry the yellow fever virus are found in many countries around the world, there is ongoing potential for the disease to be brought back in an infected traveller, thus causing new outbreaks in new areas. For this reason the countries at highest risk, particularly in Asia, require proof of immunization against the disease for anyone who enters the country from South America or Africa. Long-term travellers need to consider this risk when planning their extended trip; they should be vaccinated before they leave home if they plan on travelling in or through the endemic areas of South America or Africa.

## Japanese Encephalitis

The next vaccine the long-term traveller should consider is against another mosquito-borne disease called Japanese encephalitis (JE). The Japanese encephalitis virus lives in a mosquito species called *Culex*, which are also linked to the West Nile virus. JE belongs to a family of viruses called flaviviruses and was named for the area where it was first isolated. The JE virus also infects pigs and birds but generally doesn't make them sick. In humans the virus can cause severe inflammation of the brain, which can be fatal in as many as 30 percent of people who become ill. Most suffer from milder disease, but the long-term effects are devastating and can result in permanent loss of hearing and paralysis. Unlike yellow fever, this virus lives in rural areas, particularly where there is an abundance of pigs and birds, and is almost never found in urban environments. It is also a seasonal disease that is most active during the summer and fall.

The areas at risk for this bug include India, Southeast Asia, Japan, and Korea. A vaccine developed in Japan in the 1930s has largely controlled the disease in China, Korea, Japan, Taiwan, Singapore, and Thailand. Unfortunately the vaccine is costly and some countries do not have the resources to implement immunization programs against JE. Countries that continue to have sporadic outbreaks of the disease include Vietnam, Cambodia, Myanmar (Burma), India, Nepal, and Malaysia. Anyone travelling to these areas, particularly the rural parts of the country, during the risk period and are staying for longer than four weeks should consider receiving the vaccination for this disease.

## Meningitis

Another immunization that a long-term traveller should consider is vaccination against meningitis. Several effective vaccines are available for meningitis, and in many Western countries new routine immunization programs protect children from the disease. Meningitis is a general term for the infection of the lining of the brain, but the most severe forms of the disease are caused by a bacterium called *Neisseria meningitidis*. This bug belongs to the same family as *Neisseria gonorrhoeae* but is transmitted between people by respiratory droplets. Often the disease is passed from person to person through sharing of food, drink, or even cigarettes. When someone is infected with meningitis, the first signs of disease are fever, severe headache, and stiff neck with a deep purple-coloured rash. This devastating illness can lead to death or permanent disability such as deafness or paralysis.

For travellers the meningitis vaccine may be in order if they are visiting an area of the world where periodic seasonal outbreaks of this infection occur. The highest area of risk is in sub-Saharan Africa between December and June; other areas of risk include India, Nepal, and Brazil. There have also been outbreaks of meningitis in pilgrims in Saudi Arabia in recent years. In 2000 more than 250 pilgrims who travelled to Mecca to participate in the hajj developed a rare form of meningitis caused by the bacteria *Neisseria meningitidis* serogroup W-135. The three million pilgrims included some who came from countries in the African meningitis belt. Crowding, shared food and drink, and exhaustion are some of the contributing factors that make the pilgrimage conducive to the spread of infection. Public health officials traced the disease to dozens of countries, including Canada, the United States, Denmark, France, Norway, Singapore, the United Kingdom, and the entire Middle East. In some cases the disease had been passed on to other family members. Quick action by public health officials in these countries prevented more cases of disease, but tragically more than forty-five fatalities were reported. The government of Saudi Arabia has since implemented strict requirements, insisting that all pilgrims be vaccinated and even providing the vaccine at various points of entry, and turning people back who refuse the immunization.

### Typhoid and Cholera: Two Old Foes

Other vaccines the long-term traveller ought to contemplate are for protection against the now rare diseases typhoid and

cholera. Typhoid is a disease caused by the bacterium
*Salmonella typhi*, a sibling of the *Salmonella* species that induces
common gastrointestinal illness. Typhoid is an infection of
the blood that develops one to three weeks after exposure to
the bacteria and can cause mild to severe disease symptoms,
including high fever, headache, lack of appetite, diarrhea or
constipation, a rose-coloured rash that often appears on the
chest, and swelling of the liver and spleen. The disease can
be fatal in as many as 10 percent of those who are infected,
and some, like Typhoid Mary, become long-term carriers
after they have recovered, passing the bug on to others
through contaminated food. Typhoid can be treated with
antibiotics, but resistance to these medications is common in
many parts of the world, so prevention is by far the best
option.

Typhoid is spread through food and drink contaminated
with sewage. The disease was common in North America
and Europe in the 1800s but has been largely eliminated by
adequate sanitation and sewage systems. But in areas of the
world where handwashing is less frequent and sewage systems are rudimentary, the bacterium still flourishes. In Asia,
Africa, and Latin America as many as 21.5 million people
contract typhoid every year. Recently there have been dramatic outbreaks in some countries, including Haiti, where
more than two hundred cases were reported from one area of
the island in 2003 and resulted in forty deaths, and the
Democratic Republic of the Congo, where between September
2004 and January 2005 a staggering 42,564 cases were
reported to the WHO and 214 people died in the city of
Kinshasa. In the United States around four hundred cases of
typhoid are reported every year, and the vast majority are in
people who have recently travelled to a developing country.

There are two different vaccines that protect against typhoid; though neither is 100 percent effective, they are in the 70 to 90 percent range. Both need to be taken at least a week before going to a high-risk area, to allow immunity to build up, and both last only a few years, so boosters are required every two to five years. While the vaccine helps mitigate the worst symptoms of disease, it doesn't negate the need to be careful about food and water, to avoid unpasteurized milk, and to be obsessive about hand cleaning before eating and after using the toilet.

The same goes for the cholera vaccine, which offers short-term protection but is not absolute. An injectable cholera vaccine has been available for more than forty years, but it provides short-term protection only and is not recommended for travellers. The vaccine has been used on a broad scale in some countries during large outbreaks but its effectiveness is questionable and the WHO does not recommend using the vaccine. New oral vaccines are now available that offer better protection and are available in some countries, including Canada and most of Europe. These medications should be considered by long-term travellers going to areas of the world where cholera epidemics are still common.

Cholera is an acute and sometimes severe diarrheal illness caused by the bacterium *Vibrio cholerae*. In severe cases patients suffer such massive fluid loss that they can die in a matter of hours, so the most important treatment is rapid replacement of fluids. Cholera has such tremendous outbreak potential that every country around the world is required by the International Health Regulations to report outbreaks of infection immediately to the WHO. The WHO reports that more than 130,000 people are infected with cholera every year, with close to 2,300 fatalities; over 95 percent of cases are in countries in Africa and the rest are in a few countries in South America.

Unfortunately cholera is re-emerging in many countries, particularly in western Africa and most spectacularly in Zimbabwe, where between August and December 2008 11,735 cases and 484 deaths were reported to the WHO. This massive outbreak reflects the complete breakdown of the health, water, and sanitation systems of this previously rich and healthy country under the authoritarian rule of President Robert Mugabe. Unless you are travelling specifically to work in one of the highly affected areas, the risk of contracting cholera is very low. The vaccine should be an adjunct to all the other important safety measures, especially avoiding contaminated food and drink.

## Dog Bites and Death

As we saw in Chapter 1, rabies is a viral disease that attacks the nervous system and is almost universally fatal in humans. The virus that causes the disease is transmitted to humans through bites or scratches from infected animals. Throughout history the horrible effects of rabies and the slow, painful death associated with the disease has been a stimulus for scientific discovery. It was the young Louis Pasteur's experience of seeing a fellow villager die from rabies that inspired his work on the development of a vaccine. Today there are effective vaccines for animals, and bylaws across North America and Europe require that pets be immunized. As a result rabies has been largely eliminated in these areas. But the disease remains a major issue in many developing countries where vaccination of pets is not available or affordable.

In North America and Europe, rabies is a disease of warm-blooded wild animals, especially foxes, raccoons, coyotes, skunks, and bats. Human exposure is relatively rare but does happen on occasion, usually from inadvertent exposure to rabid bats that may enter houses when they are ill and bite or scratch the unsuspecting occupants. With the development of animal control and vaccination programs in the 1940s, the number of people infected with rabies in North America fell dramatically in the past century from more than a hundred cases every year to two or three cases annually. Between 1990 and 2001 thirty-six cases of rabies were reported in the United States, and one-third of the cases were in people who had contracted the disease while travelling. Most were bitten by dogs, though a monkey bite was the cause in at least one case. In the United Kingdom, twelve cases of rabies, all fatal, were reported between 1995–2009, and ten of those people were infected while visiting the Indian subcontinent. In France eighteen of the nineteen cases of rabies in that period were also related to travel.

Worldwide rabies remains a devastating and all-too-common disease, with more than fifty thousand deaths caused by the virus every year. The WHO estimates that more than half of these fatalities occur on the Indian subcontinent, where rabid dogs run wild in urban centres and rural villages. The other cases are located primarily in Africa, Latin America, and Southeast Asia, especially the Philippines and Thailand, where in Bangkok one in ten stray dogs carries the deadly infection. In 2008 there were seventeen human cases of rabies in Latin America, with dogs being the vector in Brazil, Bolivia, El Salvador, Guatemala, Argentina, and the Dominican Republic, and bats the offender in Mexico.

So who needs to be concerned about rabies before they travel? Anyone who is going to be working with animals or spending time outdoors, particularly in remote areas or in some developing countries where access to safe and effective treatment cannot be guaranteed. The vaccine for humans that protects against rabies involves a series of five shots that must be administered shortly after the person has been scratched or bitten. For those who may be at high risk of exposure or who won't have access to treatment, two shots of the protective immunization can be administered before travel. This will protect people initially and give them time to access a safe supply of vaccine for the final three shots. Children should also be considered for this pre-travel vaccine as they tend to be at higher risk of exposure because of their tendency to play with animals.

RETURNING HOME

The final group of long-term travellers are affectionately known in the business as VFRS. VFR stands for visiting friends and relatives, and refers to the large group of people who have emigrated to Western countries from developing countries. They often maintain strong family and economic ties to their home country and frequently return for extended visits. For a number of reasons this group of travellers may be at the highest risk of infection of all the groups we have considered so far. First, VFRs frequently take the whole family, including children and grandparents, on their travels back home. Visits are often for an extended period of time and may take place in rural areas, where they stay with local families and eat and drink the local food.

As we have seen, people who grow up in areas with poor drinking water and sanitation, if they survive their first few bouts of diarrheal illness, will develop some immunity against these bugs for the next few years. If, however, they move to another part of the world such as Canada or England, for example, they will lose this immunity and can become seriously ill when they travel back to their home country. So the combination of travelling in groups with family members who need special considerations and staying in rural areas with poor sanitation systems increases the possibility for VFRs to contract and spread communicable disease among family members and to others in their new home country. Let's take a look at some of the illnesses common to this group of travellers and the measures we can take to prevent contracting these diseases.

## Malaria

One major consideration for this group of travellers is the mosquito-borne disease malaria. Malaria is a severe febrile illness caused by one of four different species of the bug *Plasmodium*: *vivax, ovale, malariae,* and the most deadly one, *falciparum.* Illness is characterized by high fevers, severe muscle aches, headaches, and vomiting. Before West Nile virus appeared on the scene, it had been some time since mosquito-borne diseases were at all a concern in North America and most of Europe. While mosquito-control programs helped eliminate these deadly infections from most of the Western world, they still rank supreme on the list of lethal infections in many other parts of the globe. Malaria alone is responsible for millions of deaths worldwide every year, and it hits young children particularly hard. The disease is rampant in most of Southeast Asia, Asia, and Africa, with drug-resistant strains now the norm in many countries. Not only that, malaria and a viral mosquito-borne illness, dengue, have seen a tremendous resurgence in the past decade.

Malaria, from the Italian for "bad air," has been documented for more than four thousand years. Symptoms of the disease were written up in ancient Chinese medical writings, and it was said to be responsible for declining populations in Greece in the fourth century B.C. Ancient writings also describe using the plant quinghao, or wormwood, for treatment of fevers from malaria. Malaria was a scourge of the New World as well; in the eighteenth century explorer Simon Fraser described what is today the city of Vancouver as "nothing but a malaria-filled swamp." Spanish missionaries in South America described the decimation of towns and villages from malaria and learned of a treatment made by the indigenous tribes from the bark of a local tree. In the seventeenth century the countess of Chinchón, wife of the viceroy of Peru, was cured of her fever by a potion made from the bark of a tree that was then called Peruvian bark but later named Cinchona after the countess. The potent anti-malarial drug made from the bark of this tree is now known as quinine and is still used today.

*Plasmodium*, the parasite that causes malaria, was discovered in 1880 by French army surgeon Charles Laveran while he was stationed in Algeria. He observed the parasites in the blood of infected soldiers through the newly invented microscope, and in 1907 he was awarded the Nobel Prize for this discovery. The complex life cycle of *Plasmodium* was not worked out until much later, but its association with the illness was a key first step. After the discovery of the parasite in 1880 it was almost another two decades before British officer

Ronald Ross confirmed that mosquitoes were the vector for transmission of malaria. While he was working for the Indian Medical Service, Ross showed that the malaria parasites could be transmitted by mosquitoes that bit an infected patient, and he described transmission of the parasites between birds by mosquitoes. He won the Nobel Prize for his work in 1902.

Perhaps no other single infection has had as dramatic an impact on civilization as the scourge of malaria. The disease affected so many aspects of life, from military deployments to colonization to even the survival of cities. It was the disease's profound impact on the construction of the Panama Canal from 1905 to 1910 that led to the first successful efforts to control the disease. In 1906, 21,000 of the 26,000 workers on the canal had been hospitalized at some point for two mosquito-borne diseases, malaria and yellow fever. The rates of death from malaria were as high as sixteen of every thousand men. Because the Panama Canal was such an immense and important project, the United States could not afford to see it fail.

The government developed an intensive mosquito-control program that involved pesticides to kill adult mosquitoes, habitat destruction such as draining pools of water where mosquitoes breed, larvicide, and malaria treatment, along with liberal use of quinine to prevent illness. U.S. Medical Corps physicians William Gorgas, Joseph LePrince, and Samuel Darling spearheaded the initiative, and their work was the first large-scale undertaking to not just control but eliminate mosquito-borne disease entirely from an area. By 1912 the number of illnesses had been dramatically reduced, not only in the canal workers but also in the local population. In that year only 5,600 of more than 50,000 workers had been hospitalized for malaria, and yellow fever had been eliminated completely.

In an attempt to build on successes like those in Panama, the World Health Organization led an ambitious project in 1955 to eradicate the disease in "malarious" countries around the world. The Global Malaria Eradication Campaign used measures such as spraying infected areas with pesticides (especially DDT), treating cases with anti-malarial medication, and setting up surveillance networks in an effort to eliminate the disease for good. The initiative did succeed in eliminating malaria from most temperate countries, including much of Europe, Australia, Canada, and the United States. In addition, some countries such as India and Sri Lanka saw dramatic decreases in the numbers of illnesses and deaths from malaria.

But in much of the world where the disease was rampant, particularly sub-Saharan Africa, the gains were the least, and efforts were abandoned in 1978 in favour of control rather than eradication. The campaign had fallen victim to the survival instincts of the malaria parasite and its mosquito hosts. The mosquitoes rapidly developed resistance to the pesticides, and the malaria parasite became resistant to the medications that treat infections. Couple that with war, massive population movement, and a lack of sustained funding, and the well-meaning effort was doomed to fail.

By the time the campaign ended, malaria rates in many countries were as high as ever or even higher than before — but now there was also widespread resistance to deal with. To this day malaria remains the most important parasitic tropical disease in the world, killing more than a million people every year, which is more than any other infection except AIDS and TB. Tragically, the majority of the deaths are of children under the age of five, particularly those who live in remote areas with little or no access to medical care. In Africa one in five children (20 percent) under five years of age dies from malaria. The

WHO estimates that somewhere between 300 to 500 million people get sick from the disease every year, and most of them live in the hundred or so malaria-endemic countries. Over 40 percent of the world's population — 2.4 billion people — live in these areas, which include South America, the eastern Mediterranean, Southeast Asia, South Asia, and sub-Saharan Africa, where the most deadly strain, *P. falciparum*, reigns.

Not only are millions still affected by malaria today, but in past decades we have seen dramatic increases in the disease due to global warming and weather events such as El Niño. Global temperatures have risen on average 1 to 3 degrees Celsius in the past hundred years, and this has certainly contributed to the expansion of prime mosquito breeding grounds around the world. This in turn has provided a haven for the malaria parasite, leading to a striking resurgence of infections in humans in countries such as Haiti and Jamaica, where it had been eliminated for decades. These rising rates of infection have, not surprisingly, coincided with the dismantling of mosquito-control programs in many parts of the world when attention to malaria waned after 1978.

While children can be at high risk of severe illness and death from the infection, over time people living in malarious countries develop a relative immunity to the disease. But this immunity disappears if the individual has not been exposed for some time to the parasite that causes malaria. So many who grow up in malarious countries and then move to areas of the world where the disease is uncommon lose their immunity or may not realize the high risk of severe infection that their Western-born children face. Public health officials have been trying to get this message out to those who return to South Asia, Southeast Asia, and Africa for extended visits. Sadly, they have not had much success.

Every year hundreds of people bring malaria back with them from trips abroad. In the United States 1,564 people became ill with malaria and six people died in 2006, a slight increase over the previous few years. All of the people who became ill had picked up the disease while travelling outside the country. The most common places where people were infected were western Africa and Asia, with a small number from the Caribbean and Latin America. Over 50 percent of those who contracted the disease reported that they had travelled to visit friends and relatives; long-term missionary or volunteer work was a distant second at 9.9 percent, and tourism a modest 7 percent. A similar story plays out every year in Canada and the United Kingdom where about four hundred people in Canada and about two thousand people in the U.K. become ill after returning from travel abroad. In both countries the majority (72 percent in the U.K.) of people picked up the bug when they returned to visit family and friends in West Africa or the Indian subcontinent.

Malaria is both life-threatening and preventable, but the number of people who become ill every year after travelling to these high-risk areas highlights the fact that many are unaware of the measures that can be taken to stave off the deadly infection. The longer your stay in a country with active malaria, the higher the chances you will encounter a *Plasmodium*-carrying mosquito; and the risk goes up in rural areas. This is why VFRs and other long-term travellers are at the greatest risk, though even short-term tourists and business travellers can pick up this lethal bug if they don't take the necessary precautions. Luckily most urban areas of Southeast Asia, Central America, and South America have effective mosquito-control programs, so people staying in urban centres probably don't need to worry. It is when you venture out of the cities, especially if it is for a long time, that more careful attention is needed to prevent infection.

The first line of defence starts before you leave and involves taking a medication to prevent the malaria bug from causing infection. A number of medications are available, ranging from chloroquine, the first antibiotic for malaria, to the latest combination drug, called atovaquone/proguanil. Chloroquine was a lot like the original quinine but had fewer side effects, was a more effective treatment, and, it was soon discovered, could be given to people before they went to a malarious area to prevent infection in the first place. Unfortunately, by the 1960s malaria was showing signs of resistance to this drug in Colombia and Thailand. Drug-resistant strains of the parasite have since spread around the world and are now common in many countries.

The next step is to talk to a doctor or visit a travel clinic to find out which medication ought to be taken for the area you are visiting. This measure is particularly important to protect children and pregnant women, because they are most likely to get severe or even deadly illness if infected. Malaria can have devastating effects on both pregnant women and their unborn children, so serious consideration should be given to whether travel to high-risk areas is necessary at all. If you do decide to go, taking medication to prevent infection is far safer than taking the risk of contracting the illness itself.

Once you arrive at your destination there are a few other important protective measures to take. The mosquitoes that carry malaria are night biters and lie low during the heat of the day. So it's best to stay indoors from dusk to dawn, when the mosquitoes are active and looking for blood. In many countries mosquitoes are also active just after the rainy season, so travelling during that time of year also increases the risk of contracting the bug. When you are outside, always wear a long-sleeved shirt and full-length pants, and keep clothing loose-fitting and light coloured. And remember to use bed nets to prevent being bitten at night. Repellents help make you less attractive to mosquitoes, and the most effective and long-lasting ones contain DEET and lemon eucalyptus oil. Another good idea is to wear clothing that has been treated with permethrin, a substance that kills mosquitoes on contact; you can also get treated bed nets, which provide more protection.

## Dengue Rises

The dengue virus is another mosquito-borne bug that has re-emerged as a major threat to human health and in recent years has expanded its reach globally. Dengue fever and dengue hemorrhagic fever are human illnesses caused by infection with the dengue virus. People who are bitten by infected mosquitoes develop severe headaches, muscle aches, rash, and fever within a few days. These symptoms can last for a week, though it may take several weeks to recover fully. The bone and joint pain from dengue is so severe that the disease has been nicknamed "breakbone fever." A small proportion of those infected with dengue go on to develop internal bleeding and bleeding from their nose and gums. This hemorrhagic form of the disease can be fatal in as many as 30 percent of cases, though with supportive care deaths are usually less frequent.

The WHO estimates about 50 million people are hospitalized around the world from dengue, and about half a million suffer from dengue hemorrhagic fever every year. Since its resurgence in the 1980s dengue has caused large outbreaks of disease in thousands of people in Puerto Rico, Brazil, Venezuela,

Thailand, Malaysia, Hong Kong, Taiwan, and Singapore — areas where the infection had been virtually eliminated for many years. In addition, the disease has been found for the first time in Caribbean islands such as Barbados and the U.S. Virgin Islands, as well as in Costa Rica, Panama, and Samoa.

Dengue thrives in crowded cities and uses the highly urbanized *Aedes* mosquito species as its vector. In 2002 a major outbreak in Rio de Janeiro affected a million people, and in early 2008 more than fifty thousand cases were reported, with thirty deaths. Though dengue is uncommon in Western countries, the disease is still a small but real risk in some parts of the United States and has been introduced into the Northern Territory of Australia, likely by military forces returning from duty in East Timor. There have been at least six episodes of transmission in Texas since 1980, though the initial cases were linked to outbreaks in Mexico and Hawaii. In December 2008 an outbreak of dengue in Cairns, Australia, affected more than fifty people.

For the most part the risk of contracting dengue, especially in Europe, the United States, and Canada, is from travel. However, with global warming and increasingly complex global trade routes, it is not inconceivable that the *Aedes* species of mosquitoes will be introduced into these countries and outbreaks of dengue will start anew. These global patterns may also bring other diseases to our shores, as we have seen only too clearly with the West Nile virus invasion of North America.

## Chikungunya Again

A further warning sign of the potential effects of global warming is the re-emergence of chikungunya, another mosquito-borne virus that causes an infection similar to dengue. During the 1990s this virus adapted to live in more than one species of mosquito. As mosquito numbers climbed the virus multiplied and caused an outbreak of disease in 2005 affecting more than a quarter of a million people on the French Island of Réunion in the Indian Ocean. From there this previously obscure virus caused outbreaks affecting hundreds of thousands in several Indian states in 2006. In 2007 an infected traveller returning home to Italy unwittingly started an outbreak that affected 130 people in Ravenna, a city that was previously thought not to be at risk.

The bottom line is that mosquito-borne diseases are on the rise around the world, and with increasing global temperatures and the mass movement of people and goods, new bugs and new species of mosquitoes may soon be introduced to parts of the world where the ravages of these diseases have been previously unknown.

❁

IT CAN BE daunting to think through all the myriad ways we can become ill when travelling, but if you break down the risk by where you are going and for how long, then you can plan ahead and figure out the best ways of protecting yourself against the various divisions of Microbes Inc. Once on your way, the few simple rules around safe eating and drinking, personal hygiene and sanitation, and protection against animal or insect bites will work for just about any situation.

My own experience has shown this to be true, but these measures are not foolproof even with the best of efforts. Recently I went on a trip with some friends to Africa to climb Mount Kilimanjaro. Even though I provided advice to the gang before we left, when we reached Tanzania we were very much at the mercy of the excellent company we climbed with.

Happily, I was more than impressed with the simple measures they routinely took, which ensured that we all reached the summit healthy. The simplest and most effective provision was to offer warm water and soap every morning and evening and before every meal. Cleaning your hands regularly has been proven to be the most important thing you can do to prevent getting sick, in every place you can imagine.

A fascinating study was conducted a few years ago in two remote villages in Pakistan where the water is often contaminated and children fell ill with regularity. In one village the children were provided with plain bars of soap and encouraged to wash their hands before eating; in the other village children were left to follow their normal routines. The village that was provided with soap saw rates of illness shrink dramatically and fewer children died from diarrheal illness — all because they were given a bit of soap. This lesson was repeated with our Kili climbing group: we washed with plain soap and water and none of us suffered any illness, while our neighbouring climbers, who were not as conscientious about hand hygiene, fell ill at a way-too-frequent rate.

When I spent three months in Pakistan working with the WHO, despite washing my hands and eating carefully I still managed to pick up a nasty diarrhea bug that sidelined me for a good week. I was working in a remote area, and a few weeks later when my group reconvened in Islamabad for a meeting, we discovered that four out of seven of us had similar nasty illnesses. Being good disease detectives, we searched through our memories of who had eaten what to see if we could figure out where we had slipped up. The mystery was soon resolved: about three days before we became ill we had all taken a trip to the market to buy food for a group meal. The four of us who got sick had eaten pieces of sugar cane from a bag that one of us had bought from a market stall. The other three had eaten everything except the sugar cane. Thinking back, the person who bought the treat (not me!) described the pieces of fresh sugar cane lying on the table after they had been put through a machine to remove the hard outer shell. He remembered watching the stall owner splash water on the sugar cane to keep it fresh — water from the local tap. He didn't use a lot of water, but it was enough to make the four of us pretty ill.

Being prepared reduces the risk of becoming sick, and it can also help you when things inevitably go wrong. So along with the alcohol-based hand rub, antibiotic ointment, mosquito repellent, and condoms, add to your travel list a course of medication to treat diarrhea illness that lasts more than two to three days and some Imodium, a medication that helps stop diarrhea. Let's face it, the wonders of travel and the experience of learning about a new culture and place far outweigh the risks of getting sick — most of the time. But protecting yourself and your family first and staying healthy during the trip can make the experience all that much better. So get your immunizations, clean your hands, watch out for ice cubes, raw seafood, and salads — and enjoy yourself.

❄

HOME OR ABROAD, the divisions of Microbes Inc. are always on the lookout for people to infect to increase their numbers and ensure their dominance of the planet. The measures we can take to prevent these bugs from spreading are the same everywhere we go. Immunizations are the best way to stop infections in the first place, and using antibiotics wisely and only for infections caused by bacteria helps ensure that these disease-fighting drugs will work when we need them in the future. No matter where we are in the world, antibiotics don't work on viruses, so don't be tempted to use these drugs even if they are available and commonly used to treat every ailment. And everywhere in the world, washing your hands with plain soap and water or cleaning them with an alcohol-based hand sanitizer is the simplest and most effective way to avoid illness. The wise words of Dr. William Osler, one of the founding fathers of modern medicine, come back to us again and again: "Soap and water and common sense" really are the best disinfectants.

# TOP 10 MYTHS AND TRUTHS ABOUT BUGS

1. **MYTH**: *My immune system is healthy, so I don't need immun ization. Besides, vaccines are dangerous.*

   **TRUTH**: Vaccines work with your immune system to help you fight infection. A report of a potential link between the MMR vaccine and autism has been debunked by scientific evidence. Vaccines are safe and effective, and our best protection against many infections.

2. **MYTH**: *I can stop taking antibiotics when I start to feel better.*

   **TRUTH**: Antibiotics take time to work completely against bacterial infections. You need to take the full course you are prescribed to be sure the infection is cured, even if you are feeling better.

3. MYTH: *Antibiotics will make me better when I have a cold or the flu.*

   TRUTH: Antibiotics work only against bacteria. Most coughs, earaches, and sore throats and all colds and flus are caused by viruses. Antibiotics don't work on viruses and won't help you recover from these infections.

4. MYTH: *Over-the-counter cough and cold medications cure infections.*

   TRUTH: Medications for fevers — by themselves or in combination with decongestants, antihistamines, and cough suppressants — don't cure illness. They just help make the symptoms more bearable until your body's immune system is able to fight off the virus. They may help you feel a bit better, but you could still be infectious to others. Cough and cold medications don't work and can be dangerous in young children, so they should be avoided.

5. MYTH: *Superbugs are resistant to handwashing and cleaning.*

   TRUTH: Washing your hands or using an alcohol-based hand rub will protect you from superbugs just as well as from other bacteria and viruses. Superbugs may be resistant to some antibiotics, making infections difficult to treat, but they are still susceptible to cleaning and are helpless against good hygiene.

6. MYTH: *I don't need to worry about having a fever if it's not too high.*

   TRUTH: Even a low-grade fever is often a sign that your body is fighting an infection. If you have a fever with a cough or with vomiting and diarrhea or a rash, these can all be signs that the infection may be one that you can pass on to others. You should stay home and isolate yourself, and call your health-care provider for advice if your symptoms are worrisome.

7. MYTH: *I need to use dish soap with an antibacterial agent in it to be sure that my dishes are properly cleaned and safe to use.*

   TRUTH: Plain soaps and detergents work just fine for washing dishes and clothes, cleaning your house, or washing your hands. Antibacterial agents in soaps and detergents can lead to the development of antibiotic-resistant bugs in the environment, which can then cause hard-to-treat infections.

8. MYTH: *Organic foods are safer for me and my family.*

   TRUTH: "Organic" doesn't mean free of bugs, and in fact organic fruits and vegetables may have more risk of causing infection if they are not cleaned properly or cooked before you eat them.

9. MYTH: *Unpasteurized milk is healthier for me.*

   TRUTH: Unpasteurized milk has no health benefits over pasteurized milk, and it may put you and your family at risk of infections.

10. MYTH: *Pets such as cats and dogs are immune to infectious diseases.*

TRUTH: Household pets can carry bacteria and can get sick from many types of bacteria, viruses, and parasites. To keep yourself and your family from getting an illness from your pet, always clean your hands after playing with pets or touching their food, toys, or sleeping areas, and before preparing food.

# TOP 10 WAYS
# TO STAY HEALTHY

1. Clean your hands.
2. Cover your mouth when you cough.
3. Stay at home when you have a fever.
4. Get immunized.
5. Don't take antibiotics when you are sick with a virus.
6. Cook foods to a safe temperature (see page 150), especially meat and seafood.
7. Wash foods thoroughly, especially produce that is eaten raw.
8. Frequently clean cutting boards, counters, doorknobs, toys — any and all surfaces where bugs may linger.
9. Don't use soap or detergents with antibacterial agents.
10. Use condoms.

# NOTES

THE BOOK

I used several large, occasionally terribly technical medical texts for the basic science stuff in this book and tried to translate the concepts into words and stories the average person would understand. If you have a great desire for detailed scientific background with longer words, these are the main texts I consulted (any errors in translation are entirely my own!):

Alfred S. Evans and Philip S. Brachman, *Bacterial Infections of Humans: Epidemiology and Control*, 3rd ed. (New York: Springer, 1998).
Alfred S. Evans and Richard A. Kaslow, *Viral Infections of Humans: Epidemiology and Control*, 4th ed. (New York: Springer, 1997).
Sherwood L. Gorbach, John G. Bartlett, and Neil R. Blacklow, *Infectious Diseases*, 3rd ed. (Philadelphia: Lippincott Williams & Wilkins, 2003).

David L. Heymann, *Control of Communicable Diseases Manual*, 19th ed. (Washington, DC: American Public Health Association, 2009).

G. L. Mandell, J. E. Bennett, and R. Dolin, eds., *Principles and Practice of Infectious Disease*, 6th ed. (Philadelphia: Churchill Livingstone, 2004).

Kenrad E. Nelson and Carolyn Masters Williams, *Infectious Disease Epidemiology: Theory and Practice*, 2nd ed. (Sudbury, MA: Jones & Bartlett, 2006).

Stanley A. Plotkin, *Vaccines*, 4th ed. (Philadelphia: Elsevier Science, 2004).

Most of the detailed numbers and statistics come from the following online sources, all of which produce periodic reports of outbreaks around the world as well as official statistics (all free, and some very good reading if you are interested in disease tracking).

Centers for Disease Control and Prevention, *Morbidity and Mortality Weekly Report* (MMWR), http://www.cdc.gov/mmwr/.

World Health Organization, *The Weekly Epidemiological Record*, http://www.who.int/wer/en/index.html.

Public Health Agency of Canada (formerly Health Canada), *Canada Communicable Disease Report* (CCDR), http://www.phac-aspc.gc.ca/publicat/ccdr-rmtc/.

European Centre for Disease Control, *Eurosurveillance*, http://www.eurosurveillance.org/.

International Society for Infectious Disease, *ProMED-mail*, http://www.promedmail.org/pls/otn/f?p=2400:1000:. "The global electronic reporting system for outbreaks of emerging infectious diseases and toxins." Published free online, this is a worldwide email forum of scientists who exchange information on outbreaks.

ONE: GOOD BUGS, BAD BUGS

Ted Grant and William Osler, *This Is Our Work: The Legacy of Sir William Osler* (Pakenham, ON: 5 Span Books and Canadian Medical Association, 1994).

Quite a few books have addressed the impact of infectious diseases, especially outbreaks or epidemics, on the history of the world. For those interested in more details, two I would recommend and have consulted for all the chapters of this book are Sheldon Watts, *Epidemics and History: Disease, Power, and Imperialism* (New Haven, CT: Yale University Press, 1997) and the bestseller and Pulitzer Prize winner, Jared Diamond, *Guns, Germs and Steel: The Fates of Human Societies* (New York: W. W. Norton, 1999).

For more eloquent details on smallpox and the global eradication campaign, I recommend two great books: Jonathan B. Tucker, *Scourge: The Once and Future Threat of Smallpox* (New York: Atlantic Monthly Press, 2001), for a lively discussion of the development of vaccine and modern bioterror threats, and Michael Bliss, *Plague: A Story of Smallpox in Montreal* (Toronto: HarperCollins, 1991), for a sensational look at the impact of the disease on the social and economic life of the city and the struggles of early public health workers.

Much of the Ebola musings comes from my own experience working with the WHO to assist the Ugandan government in controlling the largest Ebola outbreak to date, in Gulu in 1999–2000. Along with reports in the MMWR and from the WHO, the most eloquent story of the emergence of the disease was written by Pulitzer Prize–winning reporter Laurie Garrett in her book *The Coming Plague: Newly Emerging Diseases in a World Out of Balance* (Toronto: Penguin, 1994). Garrett also discusses the re-emergence of cholera in South America, with the details about spread and costs coming from WHO and Pan American Health Organization (PAHO) reports.

For more information on the fascinating emergence of *Cryptococcus* in the Pacific Northwest, several research articles were published by my colleagues at the B.C. Centre for Disease Control in the January 2007 issue of *Emerging Infectious Diseases*, which can be found at http://www.cdc.gov/ncidod/EID/13/1/42.htm.

TWO: HUMANS VS. MICROBES

Many books have been written about typhoid and the plight of poor Mary Mallon. One of the most interesting, and surprisingly well written, is by celebrity chef Anthony Bourdain, *Typhoid Mary: An Urban Historical* (New York: Bloomsbury, 2001).

The story of the father of epidemiology and cholera detective John Snow is well recorded and has been published in many places from journal articles to medical textbooks. It is a story that aspiring disease detectives and public health workers (me included) learn early in their careers. There is even a John Snow Society, which is active around the world. The UCLA Department of Epidemiology has developed a great website devoted to the man, http://www.ph.ucla.edu/epi/snow.html. One recent addition to the published literature about cholera and Snow is a wonderful book that addresses the issues of the day and describes the monumental contribution of Snow's methods: Steven Johnson, *The Ghost Map: The Story of London's Most Terrifying Epidemic — and How It Changed Science, Cities, and the Modern World* (New York: Riverhead Books, 2006).

Chronicles of the development of public health services around the world are varied. Much of the history can be found in old medical journals and now often on official websites (for example, those of the WHO, PAHO, and the CDC). There are a few modern stories too. For more information I would suggest M. Kaufman, "The Germ Theory and the Early Public Health Program in the United States," *Bulletin of the History of Medicine* 23 (May–June 1948); Malcolm S. Weinstein, *Health in the City: Environmental and Behavioral Influences* (Oxford: Pergamon Press, 1980); and Laurie Garrett, *Betrayal of Trust: The Collapse of Global Public Health* (New York: Hyperion, 2000).

And if you want to get a flavour of just what epidemic intelligence is all about, Berton Roueché, an award-winning reporter for the *New Yorker*, captures it wonderfully in his book *The Medical Detectives* (New York: Truman Talley Books, 1991).

For more about Dr. Herman Biggs and other important sanitarians in the United States, see Charles V. Chapin, Hermann M. Biggs, and Joseph W. Mountin, eds., "Models for Public Health Workers," *Journal of Public Health Policy* 6, no. 3 (September 1985), 300–306, and R. Bayer, L. O. Gostin, B. Jennings, B. Steinbock, eds. *Public Health Ethics: Theory, Policy, and Practice.* New York: Oxford University Press, 2007. The quote from Dr. Herman Biggs to the Board of Health can be found in C. Winslow's book *The Life of Herman Biggs* (Philadelphia: Lea and Febiger, 1929).

Much of the information about the WHO and the EPI, especially the polio eradication program, comes from my involvement with the organization and participation in polio eradication activities for the WHO and UNICEF. There is a more detailed history of the WHO and its many programs to promote and protect health around the world on its website, www.who.int.

The story of Lady Mary Wortley Montagu and Dr. Robert Jenner is another story that is well documented in the medical literature, and I retrieved most of the details from the medical textbooks above. Other sources include F. Fenner, D. A. Henderson, I. Arita, Z. Jezek, and I. D. Ladnyi, *Smallpox and Its Eradication* (Geneva: World Health Organization, 1988) and William H. McNeil, *Plagues and Peoples* (New York: Doubleday, 1976), a definitive tome on many epidemics.

The WHO quote on the eradication of smallpox is from the Thirty-Third World Health Assembly's "Declaration of the Global Eradication of Smallpox" (Geneva: World Health Organization, 8 May 1980).

For more information on the father of bacteriology, Dr. Louis Pasteur, again there are many published medical references, and a lot of information can be found through the website of his eponymous institute, http://www.pasteur.fr/ip/easysite/go/03b-000029-049/institut-pasteur. A well-written book on Pasteur's life and accomplishments is P. Debré, *Louis Pasteur*, trans. E. Forster (Baltimore: Johns Hopkins University Press, 1994).

For more information on the polio story and the contribution of the Connaught Laboratories, visit the website http://www.healthheritage research.com/Polio-Conntact9606.html.

The story of the development of modern medications, especially antibiotics, is less well-known but appears in many different areas of the medical literature. Two books that have interesting sections on the evolution of therapeutics and the pioneering work of Paul Ehrlich are Jacalyn Duffin, *History of Medicine: A Scandalously Short Introduction* (Toronto: University of Toronto Press, 1999) and Albert Lyons and R. Joseph Petrucelli, *Medicine: An Illustrated History* (New York: Abradale Press, 1987).

The hygiene and disinfection stories are also well known in the medical world, especially among the group of professionals who work hard to keep infections and superbugs out of our hospitals. Infection-control professionals have been doggedly carrying on the work of Semmelweis and Lister for more than a hundred years now. Several of the above-mentioned medical texts contain details of the work of both these men, including the rates of infection in the wards of the Vienna General Hospital during Semmelweis's handwashing trial. If you are into the history of his work, an interesting read is Sherwood B. Nuland, *The Doctors' Plague: Germs, Childbed Fever and the Strange Story of Ignaz Semmelweis* (New York: W. W. Norton, 2003).

One of the most comprehensive and effective programs to teach children, their parents, and medical professionals about the difference between viruses and bacteria, wise use of antibiotics, and the benefits of handwashing is the "Do Bugs Need Drugs?" program. Details and information on bugs, drugs, and handwashing can be found at www.dobugsneeddrugs.org. This program was developed in Alberta by Dr. Edith Blondell-Hill and Dr. Mary Carson. It has since been implemented in British Columbia and continues to grow.

The Nobel Foundation provides information on all the Nobel Prize recipients, available at http://nobelprize.org. The Nobel museum can be accessed from this site; it has a wealth of information on past recipients of the Nobel science and medicine prizes.

THREE: BUGS IN THE AIR

The story and most of the details of the SARS outbreak in Toronto presented in this chapter come from my intimate involvement in the outbreak as one of the lead public health officials with the City of Toronto. Any inaccuracies are solely the result of my imperfect memory.

The quote from Benjamin Franklin can be found on the PBS website http://www.pbs.org/benfranklin/l3_inquiring_medical.html.

Information on the work of the Common Cold Research Unit in the United Kingdom was found at http://www.mod.uk/DefenceInternet/ AboutDefence/WhatWeDo/HealthandSafety/PortonDownVolunteers/ TheMedicalResearchCouncilCommonColdResearchUnit.htm, and on the Common Cold Centre at Cardiff University at http://www.cardiff .ac.uk/biosi/subsites/cold/.

Several other books provide more descriptive and eloquent versions of the synopsis I have given in this chapter on the common cold, influenza, TB, and diphtheria. Here are two to consider for more information and a good read: Gina Kolata, *Flu: The Story of the Great Influenza Pandemic of 1918 and the Search for the Virus That Caused It* (New York: Touchstone Publishing, 1999) and Pete Davies, *Catching Cold: The Hunt for a Killer Virus* (London: Penguin, 2000).

Information on the recent "swine" influenza outbreak comes directly from my work at the B.C. Centre for Disease Control and as a member of national and international advisory committees on the issue. The numbers are from the official WHO reports up to the first week of May 2009. There were undoubtedly many more cases, but these statistics represent the people who were tested for the virus and found to be positive by a laboratory.

Thomas Dormandy, *The White Death: A History of Tuberculosis* (New York: New York University Press, 2000).

For the Balto story, amongst others, see Alfred Bollet, *Plagues and Poxes: The Rise and Fall of Epidemic Disease* (New York: Demos Medical Publishing, 1987).

## FOUR: BUGS WE EAT AND DRINK

The opening story in this chapter was summarized in a report in the *Globe and Mail* by Canadian Press reporter Sheryl Ubelacker in September 2005 and the details were published in the CCDR in May 2006 at http://www.phac-aspc.gc.ca/publicat/ccdr-rmtc/06vol32/dr3209a-eng.php.

The data on and history of food-borne illness surveillance is from the CDC website and MMWR reports available online. In the medical literature, several summaries include D. G. Maki, "Coming to Grips with Foodborne Infection: Peanut Butter, Peppers and Nationwide Salmonella Outbreaks," *New England Journal of Medicine* 360, no. 10 (2009), 949–53; A. Akhtar, M. Greger, H. Ferdowsian, and E. Frank, "Health Professionals' Role in Animal Agriculture, Climate Change, and Human Health," *American Journal of Preventive Medicine* 36, no. 2 (2009), 182–87; and D. Moore, "Foodborne Infections," *Canadian Journal of Infectious Diseases and Medical Microbiology* 19, no. 6 (2008), 431–33. Also very thought-provoking are two books by veterinarian and epidemiologist Dr. David Waltner-Toews, *Food, Sex and Salmonella: Why Our Food Is Making Us Sick* (Vancouver: Greystone Books, 2008) and *The Chickens Fight Back: Pandemic Panics and Deadly Diseases That Jump from Animals to Humans* (Vancouver: Greystone Books, 2007).

The information on the biosecurity program in Sweden comes from a number of sources, including *Eurosurveillance* and reports from the FAO (United Nations Food and Agriculture Organization), which functions like the WHO in the food and animal world. Reports were found at http://www.fao.org/docrep/meeting/004/ab456e.htm.

The salmonella and chocolate story and the emergence of E. coli O157:H7 and the *Listeria* outbreak were also pieced together from FAO, WHO, CDC, and PHAC reports along with medical journal articles and news reports. The Walkerton story was well reported in the medical literature and is also taken from public health reports from my colleagues in Ontario, where I was working as a medical officer of health at the time of the outbreak. Details of the public inquiry into the outbreak are available online at http://www.attorneygeneral.jus.gov.on.ca/english/about/pubs/walkerton/.

The climate change report is from the WHO Intergovernmental Panel on Climate Change (IPCC), which can be found at http://www.ipcc.ch/ipccreports/tp-climate-change-water.htm.

The issue of botulism from traditional foods is one that I learned about when I returned to the West Coast in 2005. There is a report in the MMWR about the Alaskan Natives — A. Horn, K. Stamper, D. Dahlberg et al., "Botulism Outbreak Associated with Eating Fermented Food: Alaska, 2001," MMWR 50 (2001), 680–82 — and in the CCDR on the Canadian Inuit and First Nations, at www.phac-aspc.gc.ca/publicat/ccdr-rmtc/02vol28/dr2806ea.html. For more information on safe preparation of traditional foods, the Alaska State Department of Health has some excellent resources at http://www.epi.hss.state.ak.us/pubs/botulism/Botulism.pdf.

The Albert Einstein quote comes from his book The World as I See It (Houston, TX: Filiquarian Publishing, 2006).


FIVE: BUGS IN THE NEIGHBOURHOOD

The opening story in this chapter comes from reports in the MMWR and discussions with colleagues who work in public health in California. This is an area where public health has only recently ventured, and I have been involved in setting up programs in Toronto for inspection and monitoring of personal service settings. The references to the acupuncture outbreak and hepatitis B infections from tattoos in young people in Toronto come from investigations I was involved in. The accompanying U.S. statistics are from the MMWR.

The article on superbugs and hospitals was written by Coco Ballantyne for *Scientific American* (18 October 2007) and can be accessed at http://www.scientificamerican.com/article.cfm?id=hospitals-and-superbugs. Another helpful article, published in *Canadian Health* in November 2008, is "From Wonder Drugs to Superbugs," by Bonnie Schiedel, at www.canadian-health.ca.

The story of MRSA and its move into the community is reported as well in the MMWR and in several scientific papers, including http://www.cdc.gov/mmwr/preview/mmwrhtml/mm5205a4.htm; http://www.cdc.gov/mmwr/preview/mmwrhtml/mm5233a4.htm; and http://www.cdc.gov/mmwr/PDF/wk/mm4832.pdf. See also R. M. Klevens et al., "Changes in the Epidemiology of Methicillin-Resistant Staphylococcus Aureus in Intensive Care Units in U.S. Hospitals, 1992–2003," *Clinical Infectious Diseases* 42 (2006), 389–91, and M. J. Kuehnert et al., "Methicillin-Resistant Staphylococcus Aureus Hospitalizations, United States," *Emerging Infectious Diseases* 11 (2005), 868–72. In Canada I participated in a national consensus conference that addressed the issue of MRSA's move into the community, and much of the information I present comes from a report on the conference that can be found in the *Canadian Journal of Infectious Diseases and Medical Microbiology* 18, no. 1 (January/February 2007).

Information on the Quebec outbreak of *C. difficile* was found in a number of academic publications and a report from the Ministry of Health in Quebec at www.msss.gouv.qc.ca/sujets/prob_sante/nosocomiales/index.php?situation_in_quebec, as well as from discussions with colleagues across the country and in the United States.

The Maidstone and Tunsbridge Wells story was found at http://www.mtw.nhs.uk/ and was also discussed at scientific meetings with colleagues from the United Kingdom.

The *legionella* discovery story is now well documented in medical textbooks. Information on more recent outbreaks was found through the WHO, MMWR, and the European Working Group for Legionella Infections (www.ewgli.org). The story of the care home in Toronto is based on my work as part of an expert panel to review the outbreak in Toronto in 2005. An excellent story written by Lawrence K. Altman describing the discovery of the bug appeared in the *New York Times* (1 August 2006) and can be found at www.nytimes.com/2006/08/01/health/01docs .html?_r=2&oref=slogin&pagewanted=print.

While the West Nile in America story can be found in statistics and reports from the CDC, PHAC, and such websites as that of the New York City Department of Health and Mental Hygiene (www.nyc.gov/html/ doh/html/wnv/wnvhome.shtml), much of the detail comes from my own work in Ontario and British Columbia as the virus moved across the country.

Summaries of outbreaks in recreational water sources are available at the CDC website, in their MMWR supplemental reports (www.cdc.gov/ mmwr/preview/mmwrhtml/ss5709a1.htm).

The American Pet Products Manufacturers website has a host of information on pets in homes in North America, and the results of its National Pet Owners Survey are easily accessible online at www.americanpetproducts.org/press_industrytrends.asp. I have summarized the stories of salmonella and turtles, pet treat outbreaks, exotic pets, and the monkey pox outbreak from details found in several medical publications and epidemiological reports, as well as my own experience. A nice MMWR summary of the monkey pox outbreak can be found at www.cdc.gov/mmwr/preview/mmwrhtml/mm5223a1.htm. Updates are available at the same site, along with information for pet owners and suppliers.

The *E. coli* outbreak in the petting zoo in London, Ontario, was one of my first outbreak investigations. It was published with my colleagues, particularly Dr. Bryna Warshawsky, the medical officer of health in London, who led the investigation. If you are interested in the details see B. Warshawsky, I. Gutmanis, B. Henry, et al., "An Outbreak of *Escherichia coli* O157:H7 Related to Animal Contact at a Petting Zoo," *Canadian Journal of Infectious Diseases and Medical Microbiology* 13, no. 3 (2002), 175–81. Other reports that followed are documented in the

MMWR and *Eurosurveillance* as well as in public health reports in Canada, the United States, and the United Kingdom.

## SIX: TRAVEL BUGS

One of the nicest summaries of travel-related infections comes from the *New England Journal of Medicine* of a few years ago, written by some of the leading Canadian experts on the subject (some of whom I consult regularly!): E. T. Ryan, M. Wilson, and K. Kain, "Illness after International Travel," *New England Journal of Medicine* 347, no. 7 (2002), 505–16. Other information on outbreaks in various countries comes from the WHO and CDC and is supplemented by my own experiences, especially in the case of the hepatitis A outbreak in Toronto.

The section on sexually transmitted infections comes mainly from the medical texts cited but is supplemented by a number of excellent books and papers, including Alfred S. Kaplan, ed., *The Herpes Viruses* (New York: Academic Press, 1973); Theodor Rosebury, *Microbes and Morals* (New York: Ballantine, 1973); and B. Roizman and R. J. Whitley, "The Nine Ages of Herpes Simplex Virus," *Herpes* 8, no. 1 (2001), 23–27. See also Randy Shilts, *And the Band Played On: Politics, People and the AIDS Epidemic* (New York: St. Martin's Press, 1987). The movie *And the Band Played On*, starring Matthew Modine and Alan Alda, is based on this award-winning book.

As in the other chapters, I relied heavily on the WHO and CDC for statistics on rates of disease and supplemented these stats with information from medical texts and histories available on the CDC website, particularly for yellow fever and malaria control. An interesting factual read about mosquitoes is found in Gordon Harrison, *Mosquitoes, Malaria and Man: A History of Hostilities Since 1880* (New York: Dutton, 1978).

The handwashing study in Pakistan was published in the *Journal of the American Medical Association*: S. P. Luby, M. Agboatwalla, J. Painter, A. Altaf, W. Billhimer, and R. M. Hoekstra, "Effect of Intensive Handwashing Promotion on Childhood Diarrhea in High-Risk Communities in Pakistan: A Randomized Controlled Trial," *JAMH* 291, vol. 21 (2 June 2004), 2547–54. It has since been repeated in refugee communities in Karachi, with similar positive effects. Sometimes simple works.

The book that has so far most influenced my observations during my work trying to control epidemics around the world was written not about infectious disease but about human behaviour in times of duress. It is Albert Camus' book *The Plague*, translated by Robin Buss (London: Allen Lane, Penguin Press, 2001). It was first published as *La peste* in 1947. In it he writes: "All I can say is that on this earth there are pestilences and victims — and as far as possible one must refuse to be on the side of the pestilence." I hope in some small way this book helps guide you away from the side of the pestilence.

# FURTHER
# READING

BOOKS, JOURNALS, NEWSPAPERS, MAGAZINES

Akhtar, A., M. Greger, H. Ferdowsian, and E. Frank. "Health
Professionals' Role in Animal Agriculture, Climate Change, and
Human Health." *American Journal of Preventive Medicine* 36, no. 2
(2009): 182–87.
Altman, Lawrence K. "In Philadelphia 30 Years Ago, an Eruption of
Illness and Fear." *New York Times*, August 1, 2006. http://www
.nytimes.com/2006/08/01/health/01docs.html?_r=3&oref=slogin
&pagewanted=print.
Ballantyne, Coco. "Hospitals and Superbugs: Go in Sick…Get Sicker."
*Scientific American*, 18 October 2007. http://www.scientificamerican
.com/article.cfm?id=hospitals-and-superbugs.
Bliss, Michael. *Plague: A Story of Smallpox in Montreal*. Toronto:
HarperCollins, 1991.

Bollet, Alfred. *Plagues and Poxes: The Rise and Fall of Epidemic Disease.*
New York: Demos Medical Publishing, 1987.

Bourdain, Anthony. *Typhoid Mary: An Urban Historical.* New York:
Bloomsbury, 2001.

Camus, Albert. *The Plague.* Translated by Robin Buss. London: Allen
Lane, Penguin Press, 2001.

*Canadian Journal of Infectious Diseases and Medical Microbiology* 18,
no. 1 (January/February 2007).

Chapin, Charles V., Hermann M. Biggs, and Joseph W. Mountin, eds.
"Models for Public Health Workers." *Journal of Public Health Policy*
6, no. 3 (September 1985): 300–06.

Davies, Pete. *Catching Cold: The Hunt for a Killer Virus.* London:
Penguin, 2000.

Debré, P. *Louis Pasteur.* Translated by E. Forster. Baltimore: Johns
Hopkins University Press, 1994.

Diamond, Jared. *Guns, Germs and Steel: The Fates of Human Societies.*
New York: W. W. Norton, 1999.

Dormandy, Thomas. *The White Death: A History of Tuberculosis.* New
York: New York University Press, 2000.

Duffin, Jacalyn. *History of Medicine: A Scandalously Short Introduction.*
Toronto: University of Toronto Press, 1999.

Einstein, Albert. *The World As I See It.* Houston, TX: Filiquarian
Publishing, 2006.

Evans, Alfred S., and Philip S. Brachman. *Bacterial Infections of
Humans: Epidemiology and Control,* 3rd ed. New York: Springer,
1998.

Evans, Alfred S., and Richard A. Kaslow. *Viral Infections of Humans:
Epidemiology and Control,* 4th ed. New York: Springer, 1997.

Fenner, F., D. A. Henderson, I. Arita, Z. Jezek, and I. D. Ladnyi.
"Smallpox and Its Eradication." Geneva: World Health
Organization, 1988.

Garrett, Laurie. *Betrayal of Trust: The Collapse of Global Public Health.*
New York: Hyperion, 2000.

————. *The Coming Plague: Newly Emerging Diseases in a World
Out of Balance.* Toronto: Penguin, 1994.

Gorbach, Sherwood L., John G. Bartlett, and Neil R. Blacklow. *Infectious Diseases*, 3rd ed. Philadelphia: Lippincott Williams & Wilkins, 2003.

Grant, Ted, and William Osler. *This Is Our Work: The Legacy of Sir William Osler*. Pakenham, ON: 5 Span Books and Canadian Medical Association, 1994.

Harrison, Gordon. *Mosquitoes, Malaria and Man: A History of Hostilities Since 1880*. New York: Dutton, 1978.

Heymann, David L., ed. *Control of Communicable Diseases Manual*, 19th ed. Washington, DC: American Public Health Association, 2008.

Horn, A., K. Stamper, D. Dahlberg, et al. "Botulism Outbreak Associated with Eating Fermented Food: Alaska, 2001." MMWR 50 (2001): 680–82.

Johnson, Steven. *The Ghost Map: The Story of London's Most Terrifying Epidemic — and How It Changed Science, Cities, and the Modern World*. New York: Riverhead Books, 2006.

Kaplan, Alfred S., ed. *The Herpes Viruses*. New York: Academic Press, 1973.

Kaufman, M. "The Germ Theory and the Early Public Health Program in the United States." *Bulletin of the History of Medicine* 22 (May–June 1948).

Klevens, R. M., et al. "Changes in the Epidemiology of Methicillin-Resistant Staphylococcus Aureus in Intensive Care Units in U.S. Hospitals, 1992–2003." *Clinical Infectious Diseases* 42 (2006): 389–91.

Kolata, Gina. *Flu: The Story of the Great Influenza Pandemic of 1918 and the Search for the Virus That Caused It*. New York: Touchstone, 1999.

Kuehnert, M. J., et al. "Methicillin-Resistant Staphylococcus Aureus Hospitalizations, United States." *Emerging Infectious Diseases* 11 (2005): 868–72.

Luby, S. P., M. Agboatwalla, J. Painter, A. Altaf, W. Billhimer, and R. M. Hoekstra. "Effect of Intensive Handwashing Promotion on Childhood Diarrhea in High-Risk Communities in Pakistan: A Randomized Controlled Trial." *Journal of the American Medical Association* 291, no. 21 (2 June 2004): 2547–54.

Lyons, Albert, and R. Joseph Petrucelli. *Medicine: An Illustrated History*. New York: Abradale Press, 1987.

Maki, D. G. "Coming to Grips with Foodborne Infection: Peanut Butter, Peppers and Nationwide Salmonella Outbreaks." *New England Journal of Medicine* 360, no. 10 (2009): 949–53.

Mandell, G. L., J. E. Bennett, and R. Dolin, eds. *Principles and Practice of Infectious Disease*, 6th ed. Philadelphia: Churchill Livingstone, 2004.

McNeil, William H. *Plagues and Peoples.* New York: Doubleday, 1976.

Moore, D. "Foodborne Infections." *Canadian Journal of Infectious Diseases and Medical Microbiology* 19, no. 6 (2008): 431–33.

Mtitka, M. "200 Years of Protecting the Public Health." *Journal of the American Medical Association* 280, no. 7 (19 August 1998): 592.

Nelson, Kenrad E., and Carolyn Masters Williams. *Infectious Disease Epidemiology: Theory and Practice*, 2nd ed. Sudbury, MA: Jones & Bartlett, 2006.

Nuland, Sherwood B. *The Doctors' Plague: Germs, Childbed Fever and the Strange Story of Ignaz Semmelweis.* New York: W. W. Norton, 2003.

Plotkin, Stanley A. *Vaccines*, 4th ed. Philadelphia: Elsevier Science, 2004.

Roizman, B., and R. J. Whitley. "The Nine Ages of Herpes Simplex Virus." *Herpes* 8, no. 1 (2001): 23–27.

Rosebury, Theodor. *Microbes and Morals.* New York: Ballantine, 1973.

Rouché, Berton. *The Medical Detectives.* New York: Truman Talley Books, 1991.

Ryan, E. T., M. Wilson, and K. Kain. "Illness after International Travel." *New England Journal of Medicine* 347, no. 7 (2002): 505–16.

Schiedel, Bonnie. "From Wonder Drugs to Superbugs." *Canadian Health*, November 2008. http://www.canadian-health.ca/2_6/38_e.html.

Shift, Randy. *And the Band Played On: Politics, People and the AIDS Epidemic.* New York: St. Martin's Press, 1987.

Spielman, A., and M. D'Antonio. *Mosquito: A Natural History of our Most Persistent and Deadly Foe.* New York, Hyperion, 2001.

Tucker, Jonathan B. *Scourge: The Once and Future Threat of Smallpox.* New York: Atlantic Monthly Press, 2001.

Ubelacker, Sheryl. "Bear Meat Bites Back." *Globe and Mail*, September 28, 2005. http://www.theglobeandmail.com/servlet/story/RTGAM.20050928.wbearz0928/BNStory/specialScience andHealth/.

Waltner-Toews, David. *The Chickens Fight Back: Pandemic Panics and Deadly Diseases That Jump from Animals to Humans.* Vancouver: Greystone Books, 2007.

—. *Food, Sex, and Salmonella: Why Our Food Is Making Us Sick.* Vancouver: Greystone Books, 2008.

Warshawsky, B., I. Gutmanis, B. Henry, J. Dow, J. Reffle, G. Pollett, R. Ahmed, J. Aldom, D. Alves, A. Chagla, B. Ciebin, F. Kolbe, F. Jamieson, and F. Rodgers. "An Outbreak of *Escherichia coli* O157:H7 Related to Animal Contact at a Petting Zoo." *Canadian Journal of Infectious Diseases and Medical Microbiology* 13, no. 3 (2002): 175–81.

Watts, Sheldon. *Epidemics and History: Disease, Power, and Imperialism.* New Haven, CT: Yale University Press, 1997.

Weinstein, Malcolm S. *Health in the City: Environmental and Behavioral Influences.* Oxford: Pergamon Press, 1980.

WEBSITES

Alaska State Department of Health on safe preparation of traditional foods: http://www.epi.hss.state.ak.us/pubs/botulism/Botulism.pdf

American Pet Products Manufacturers and its National Pet Owners Survey: www.americanpetproducts.org/press_industrytrends.asp

Canadian Coalition for Immunization Awareness and Promotion, for accurate, credible information on immunization: www.immunize.ca

*Cryptococcus gattii* information in *Emerging Infectious Diseases* (January 2007): http://www.cdc.gov/ncidod/EID/13/1/42.htm

*Canadian Communicable Disease Report* (CCDR), Public Health Agency of Canada (formerly Health Canada): http://www.phac-aspc.gc.ca/publicat/ccdr-rmtc/

CCDR on trichinellosis: http://www.phac-aspc.gc.ca/publicat/ccdr-rmtc/06vol32/dr3209a-eng.php

*Canadian Health Magazine*: www.canadian-health.ca

Common Cold Centre at Cardiff University: http://www.cardiff.ac.uk/biosi/subsites/cold/

Do Bugs Need Drugs? program: www.dobugsneeddrugs.org

European Working Group for Legionella Infections: www.ewgli.org
*Eurosuveillance*, European Centre for Disease Prevention and Control:
    http://ecdc.europa.eu/
Food and Agriculture Organization, United Nations, on the biosecur-
    ity program in Sweden: http://www.fao.org/docrep/meeting/004/
    ab456e.htm
Health Heritage Research Services on the polio story and the contribution
    of the Connaught Laboratories: http://www.healthheritageresearch
    .com/ Polio-Conntact9606.html
John Snow Society: http://www.johnsnowsociety.org/
*Journal of the American Medical Association*: http://jama.ama-assn.org/
Maidstone and Tunsbridge Wells NHS Trust: http://www.mtw.nhs.uk/
*Morbidity and Mortality Weekly Report* (MMWR), Centers for Disease
    Control and Prevention: http://www.cdc.gov/mmwr/
MMWR on the monkey pox outbreak: www.cdc.gov/mmwr/preview/
    mmwrhtml/mm5223a1.htm
MMWR on MRSA and its move into the community:
    http://www.cdc.gov/mmwr/preview/mmwrhtml/mm5205a4.htm
    http://www.cdc.gov/mmwr/preview/mmwrhtml/mm5233a4.htm
    and
    http://www.cdc.gov/mmwr/PDF/wk/mm4832.pdf
MMWR on outbreaks in recreational water sources: www.cdc.gov/
    mmwr/preview/mmwrhtml/ss5709a1.htm
*New England Journal of Medicine*: http://content.nejm.org/
New York City Department of Health and Mental Hygiene on West
    Nile virus: www.nyc.gov/html/doh/html/wnv/wnvhome.shtml
Nobel Foundation: http://nobelprize.org
Ontario Ministry of the Attorney General on the Walkerton tragedy:
    http://www.attorneygeneral.jus.gov.on.ca/english/about/pubs/
    walkerton/
Pasteur Institute: http://www.pasteur.fr/ip/easysite/go/03b-
    00002j-000/en
PBS on Benjamin Franklin: http://www.pbs.org/benfranklin/l3_
    inquiring_medical.html
*ProMED-mail*, International Society for Infectious Diseases:
    www.isid.org/ and www.promedmail.org

Public Health Agency of Canada (PHAC): http://www.phac-aspc.gc.ca/
PHAC on botulism outbreaks among First Nations and Inuit
communities: www.phac-aspc.gc.ca/publicat/ccdr-rmtc/02vol28/
dr2806ea.html

Quebec Ministry of Health report on the C. difficile outbreak:
www.msss.gouv.qc.ca/sujets/prob_sante/nosocomiales/index.php?
situation_in_quebec

UCLA Department of Epidemiology on John Snow: http://www.ph.ucla.
edu/epi/snow.html

United Kingdom Ministry of Defence on the Common Cold Research
Unit: http://www.mod.uk/DefenceInternet/AboutDefence/
WhatWeDo/HealthandSafety/PortonDownVolunteers/
TheMedicalResearchCouncilCommonColdResearchUnit.htm

United States Centers for Disease Control and Prevention:
http://www.cdc.gov/

Weekly Epidemiologic Record, World Health Organization:
http://www.who.int/en/

World Health Organization (WHO): www.who.int

WHO Intergovernmental Panel on Climate Change: http://www.ipcc.ch/
ipccreports/tp-climate-change-water.htm

# PERMISSIONS

John Snow's cholera map on page 35 is provided by UCLA's Department of Epidemiology in the School of Public Health. http://www.ph.ucla.edu/epi/snow

The "How Do Flu Pandemics Occur?" chart on page 86 is provided by the WHO/Western Pacific Region-Home.

The guidelines for safe cooking temperatures on page 150 are provided by the Public Health Agency of Canada and the Canadian Food Inspection Agency.

# ACKNOWLEDGEMENTS

FIRST, I WOULD like to thank House of Anansi Press, especially Sarah MacLachlan, who got me into this whole business in the first place, and to my ever so gently demanding editor Janie Yoon, who efficiently channelled my creative energy. And of course to my amazing publisher Lynn Henry, who has put up with all my stories over the years. This book would never have come to fruition without her guidance. You are brilliant; thank you.

Thank you to my many colleagues and partners in preventing pestilence who continue to support, inspire, and challenge me: especially Linda Hill, Monika Naus, Elizabeth Rea, Brain Schwartz, Marco Vittiglio, David Patrick, Ian Gemmill, Mary Vearncombe, Allison McGeer, Jim Young, and too many others to mention them all by name. I have truly been blessed to have learned from and worked with the best. Thank you to my friends and colleagues at Toronto Public Health: "common suffering builds strong bonds," and we have been through much. Thank you to the incredible team I work with at the B.C. Centre for Disease Control: you inspire me daily. Also, thank you to the grad students at the UBC School of Population and Public Health who teach me as much as I teach them, as well as the residents and field epidemiologists I have had the privilege to supervise and work with; I have learned so much from you all. No book like this can be 100 percent accurate or complete, and I am solely responsible for any errors that may have resulted from my own interpretation of science and events and for the many omissions.

Also thanks to my dear friends who have listened to my many public health rants and helped me stay real, especially Spencer Massie, and my marathon-running buddies Andrée Legendre and Ruth Conroy.

parasites, 23–26; discovery of, 45;
and food-borne diseases, 136–
41; size and character of, 26.
*See also* mosquitoes, diseases
transmitted by
parasites (specific):
*Cryptosporidium*, 173, 175–76;
*Cyclospora*, 112, 139–41;
*Giardia*, 24, 174, 183, 194;
*Trichinella*, 110–11, 112, 137–39
Parker, Janet, 44
Pasteur, Louis, 45–48; and anthrax
vaccine, 46–47; and chicken
cholera vaccine, 46; and germ
theory, 45, 57, 68, 70; and
pasteurization, 45, 100, 128–
29; and rabies vaccine, 45–46,
47–48, 56, 217
Pasteur Institute, 48; and
discovery of HIV, 202–3
Pauling, Linus, 78
pedicures, 151–52, 164–65, 166–67
penicillin, 21; discovery/
improvement of, 60–63; and
gonorrhea, 197; resistance
to, 64–65, 153, 197; and
syphilis, 200
personal service settings, 151–52,
164–67
pertussis (whooping cough) vaccine,
48, 49, 55, 56, 189, 209
Peru, 19–20, 22–23, 221
pets and animals. *See* exotic
animals and household pets
petting zoos and animal farms,
182–84
*Phytophthora infestans* (potato
blight), 22–23
plague (Black Death), 31; vaccine
for, 48, 56

plants, overbreeding of, 23
*Plasmodium*: discovery of, 221; and
mosquitoes as vector, 222,
225; *P. falciparum* (malaria
parasite), 25–26, 220
pneumococcus vaccine, 55, 56
pneumonia, 17, 31, 63, 80, 88, 197;
and HIV/AIDS, 13, 202; and
*Legionella*, 162, 163; and SARS,
94, 96; and *Staphylococcus*, 17,
66; *Streptococcus pneumoniae*,
59–60; and swine flu, 11, 89;
and tuberculosis, 100
polio, 49–55; epidemics of, 50–51;
famous sufferers, 51; and
immunization program,
52–55; occasional
re-emergence of, 54–55;
vaccine for, 49, 51–53, 56, 208
pork, *Trichinella* in, 137–38
potato blight, and Irish famine
(1845–49), 22–23
poultry, and avian flu, 85–87, 115.
*See also* avian (bird) flu
poultry and eggs: *Campylobacter* in,
120, 121–22; *Salmonella* in,
115–17
prontosil (antibiotic/sulpha
drug), 60
*Pseudomonas aeruginosa*, and hot
tub infections, 174
psittacosis ("parrot fever"), 181
public buildings, 161–64; and
*Legionella*, 162–64
public health, 32–39; and epidemiology, 33–36; and name-based
reporting, 37–38; WHO's role in,
38–39; and worldwide disease
tracking, 36–38
puerperal fever, 67–68

272 · DR. BONNIE HENRY

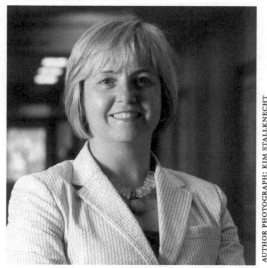

DR. BONNIE HENRY is a public health physician, a preventative medicine specialist, and an epidemiologist currently serving as the provincial health officer for British Columbia. Previously, she was the director of Public Health Emergency Management at the B.C. Centre for Disease Control and an associate medical officer at Toronto Public Health, where she was operational lead in the response to the SARS outbreak. She was also a consultant to the WHO during the 2001 Ebola outbreak in Uganda and on the STOP Polio eradication program in Pakistan, and she helped coordinate the response to the 2009 North American H1N1 pandemic. Dr. Henry is board-certified by the American College of Preventive Medicine, and she graduated from Dalhousie Medical School and completed a master's degree in Public Health from the University of California, San Diego.